The Residency Handbook

Dedication

To: Gerald Fitzgerald, M.H.A.
        President, Oakwood Health Services
        Dearborn, Michigan

whose creativity and vision has helped redefine medical education in the community hospital.

THE CLINICAL HANDBOOK SERIES

The Residency Handbook

Lyle D. Victor M.D.

Director, Transitional Residency
Oakwood Hospital
Dearborn, Michigan

and

Clinical Assistant Professor of Medicine
Wayne State University School of Medicine
Detroit, Michigan

The Parthenon Publishing Group
International Publishers in Medicine, Science & Technology

NEW YORK   LONDON

Published in the USA and Canada by:
The Parthenon Publishing Group Inc.
One Blue Hill Plaza, PO Box 1564, Pearl River, NY 10965

Published in the Europe by:
The Parthenon Publishing Group Ltd.
Casterton Hall, Carnforth, Lancs, LA6 2LA, UK

Library of Congress Cataloging-in-Publication Data
The residency handbook/(edited by) Lyle D. Victor.
   p. cm. — (The Clinical handbook series).
   Includes bibliographical references and index.
   ISBN 1-85070-583-6.
   1. Residents (Medicine) — Handbooks, manuals, etc. I. Victor,
Lyle D. II. Series.
   [DNLM: 1. Internship and Residency — organization & administration.
W 20 R4328 1994].
RA972.R45 1994.
610'.71'55 — dc20.
DNLM/DLC
for Library of Congress   94-34495
                                                                     CIP

ISBN 1-85070-583-6

Printed and bound in the USA

Contents

List of contributors

Gail Bagale, MSW
Department of Medical Education
Family Practice Residency Program Faculty
Oakwood Hospital
18101 Oakwood Boulevard
Dearborn
Michigan 48124 2500
USA

Troy R. Child, MD
Transitional Resident
Oakwood Hospital
18101 Oakwood Boulevard
Dearborn
Michigan 48124 2500
USA

Donna Craig, RN, JD
Corporation Director of Risk Management
Oakwood Hospital
18101 Oakwood Boulevard
Dearborn
Michigan 48124 2500
USA

John Escott, MD
Interim Director
Family Practice Residency Program
Oakwood Hospital
18101 Oakwood Boulevard
Dearborn
Michigan 48124 2500
USA

Stephen D. Fabick, EdD
Psychologist, Private Practice
250 Martin Street
Suite 209
Birmingham
Michigan 48009-1166
USA

Daniel D. Hendee, MSHA
Administrative Manager
Department of Medical Education
Oakwood Hospital
18101 Oakwood Boulevard
Dearborn
Michigan 48124 2500
USA

Balpreet S. Jammu, MD
Wayne State University School of Medicine
Detroit
Michigan 48214
USA

Raphael J. Kiel, MD, FACP
Associate Director
Internal Medicine Residency Program
Oakwood Hospital
18101 Oakwood Boulevard
Dearborn
Michigan 48124 2500
USA

Ronald A. Krol, EdD
Associate Director of Medical Education
Oakwood Hospital
18101 Oakwood Boulevard
Dearborn
Michigan 48124 2500
USA

Stanley Miller, MD
Assistant Director of Internal Medicine
    Residency
Oakwood Hospital
18101 Oakwood Boulevard
Dearborn
Michigan 48124 2500
USA

Sharon A. Phillips, MSLS
Director of Library and Conference
    Services
Oakwood Hospital
18101 Oakwood Boulevard
Dearborn
Michigan 48124 2500
USA

Ravi Reddy, MD
Chief Resident
Transitional Year Residency
Oakwood Hospital
18101 Oakwood Boulevard
Dearborn
Michigan 48124 2500
USA

Michelle B. Riba, MD
Assistant Clinical Professor
Department of Psychiatry
University of Michigan Medical
  Center
1500 E. Medical Center Drive
Ann Arbor
Michigan 48109
USA

**Krishna K. Sawhney,
  MB, BS, FRCS, FACS**
Chief of Surgery
Downriver Region
Henry Ford Health System
Clinical Associate Professor of
  Surgery
Wayne State School of
  Medicine
24555 Haig Taylor
Detroit
Michigan 48180
USA

Pamela E. Sawhney, RN, JD
Private Practice Law
28660 Millbrook
Farmington Hills
Michigan 48334
USA

James C. Sunstrum, MD
Clinical Assistant Professor
Wayne State University School of
  Medicine
1934 Monroe
Dearborn
Michigan 48124
USA

Dean A. Victor, DDS, CFP
Private Practice
25631 Gratiot Avenue
Roseville
Michigan 48066
USA

Lyle D. Victor, MD, FACP, FCCP
Director, Transitional Residency
Oakwood Hospital
18101 Oakwood Boulevard
Dearborn
Michigan 48124 2500
USA

Michael H. Yurkanin, MD
Transitional Resident
Oakwood Hospital
18101 Oakwood Boulevard
Dearborn
Michigan 48124 2500
USA

Foreword

While the residency is typically a rewarding period of professional preparation and personal growth, it can also be quite stressful. The resident physician must adjust to a new role and frequently, to a new environment, while coping with long hours, conflicting demands and weighty responsibility. Managing debt from medical education can add to the pressure, particularly if the resident is starting a family at the same time he or she is launching a professional career. People who choose medicine tend to be high achievers and may not have learned during medical school how to balance work and personal life. Health care professionals sometimes lack the insight to realize that they must first take care of themselves in order to take care of their patients.

In *The Residency Handbook* Dr Victor has assembled a practical guide for managing the pressure and stresses of the residency. This book offers medical students and house officers a set of 'survival skills' that will help them make a smooth transition from medical student to resident to successful professional. I recommend it highly to physicians-in-training as well as to their spouses or significant others.

Giles G. Bole, MD
Dean
University of Michigan

Preface

A physician's success is based on character and intelligence. During residency training, many qualities defining the nature of a physician's character will be discovered and developed, marking the residency years as a period of great personal and professional growth.

The Residency Handbook is written for senior medical students and junior house officers as an introduction to the special challenges of the residency training years. Medical students will appreciate the chapter on the application and interview process. Junior house officers will find the chapters on practical aspects of starting the residency training years, such as renting an apartment, starting a new job, strategies for surviving on little sleep and emotional survival, appealing. International medical graduates will find a chapter devoted to their special problems useful. More senior house officers will be interested in the chapters on financial planning and the transition to practice.

The book presents information covering many difficulties that one may encounter in the beginning of any new job...with a focus on issues particular to residency training. After reading *The Residency Handbook*, the resident will have a better understanding of the preparations, expectations and attitudes that identify the successful professional.

Lyle D. Victor

Acknowledgements

Grateful appreciation to the following individuals for their assistance in preparing this manuscript. Project co-ordination, Janelle Rose; manuscript preparation, Mary A. Hayden, Patricia Gratz and Anne Patton.

1

The application and interview process

R. Reddy and R. A. Krol

DECIDING WHERE TO APPLY

The time of your residency will mark the most important years of your professional life. Not only will you more clearly define your ultimate role as a physician but you will undergo much personal growth as well. Your first challenge will be to get the best residency possible. How you approach your residency application and interview may well determine the quality of the training program that accepts you.

The following chapter will give you an organized approach to the application and interview process by selecting key areas that are important in the medical student's and program director's selection process. Topics to be covered include: how to select a program, completing the application, interview etiquette and interview questions. Many of the interview techniques to follow may be used with modification for just about any job interview situation.

Research about what is important to medical students as they make their final choice of residency training programs indicates that while the quality and reputation of the program is an important factor, personal factors and proximity to a support system such as family are often the critical variables in the final decision. An additional factor in residency selection is a desirable geographic location[1]. This concern, however, is somewhat minimized in the more competitive specialties. Residency training can be a stressful period so you need to examine your own values and coping mechanisms to determine how high geographic and family proximity should be on your list.

If you feel that your grades, board scores and experience will give you a high probability of being accepted at a number of programs, the next step will be to evaluate the competitiveness of the programs. A technique that works is to classify programs into three groups. Group one is the highly competitive residency, group two is the moderately competitive residency and group three is the least competitive. If you believe your credentials will gain you entry to any program in the country you will probably want to interview at programs that mostly fall in the highly competitive category. However, if you feel that your grades and board scores are marginal for the specialty you are seeking, the probability of a successful match is enhanced if your pick programs for the least competitive group. The point is, if you just pick programs from the most competitive group and one ranks you lower on their list, the others may also rank you lower and you may not match. All of the most competitive use similar criteria in the selection process.

A risky strategy tried by some medical students is to only rank the most competitive programs and risk not matching, the thought being to pick up a program after the match. This is generally a poor strategy because you might be left scrambling for undesirable programs. It is in your best interest to pick a number of good programs for which you have a reasonable chance of matching.

Another concern of most students is how will you finance the expenses associated with the interviewing process. Only you can determine how much you are willing to pay to find the best program. If you are applying for highly competitive residencies you will need to find a way to travel and to interview at 10–15 programs. This can be a very expensive process indeed. It is best to construct a written travel budget in concert with your preliminary list of desired programs to determine the total budget reflected by your initial selections. Many students may need to borrow some money to finance their search for the ideal residency.

If you are granted an interview it is wise to ask if any of your interviewing expenses will be paid for. Many programs will pay for meals during the interview, some will provide lodging, and there are some programs that pay partial travel costs. The program secretary or co-ordinator is the best source of information on interviewing costs.

When you are getting ready to go on your interview you should construct a list of the criteria that are most important to you in selecting a program. You will want to find a program that has a high quality educational program and that you find as an enjoyable place to learn. These are some of the criteria you should consider.

What is the success rate of the program in the national residency matching program?
Success is a relative term with regard to the match process. The highly competitive programs such as orthopedics, radiology and obstetrics/gynecology virtually all fill their positions in the match, while the primary care programs have a fill rate of 60–80% in the match. There are regional differences that need to be taken into consideration as well. Look for a program that fills at or above the national average with highly qualified candidates. Although this usually will mean a program populated with residents having high academic credentials, some residency applicants consider the medical schools of origin important, the perception being that a program that fills with graduates of American medical schools would be preferable to a program which fills with a high percentage of international medical graduates.

What is the overall satisfaction of residents in the program?
The answer to this question will come from your interviews with residents. How satisfied do the residents feel with their training? Ask several residents this same question, understanding that, typically, the residents selected to participate in recruiting are the most satisfied residents. You should also attempt to evaluate the seriousness of the dissatisfaction. Is it with the quality of the hospital food or the lack of teaching provided?

What is the quality of the overall educational experience?
Quality in residency training is defined by many people in many ways. Most people would agree that you are looking for a program that has an organized curriculum and teaching process, as well as faculty who dedicate a significant proportion of their time to teaching. Quality for you should be defined as the program that can make you acquire the knowledge and skills you need to practice before you graduate. If residents are also treated as colleagues you may have found an ideal program for an adult learner.

What is the quality of teaching?
In the residency training process, teachers are the most significant variable in your development. This means you need to ask the residents their opinion about the quality of the teachers. Are the teachers knowledgeable? Do they use the literature to teach? Are they enthusiastic about teaching? Are they prepared? Is teaching important to them? Do they treat the residents with respect?

What is the quality of conferences?

Conferences are an integral part of any organized educational process. A well developed conference program will help enhance your training needs by giving you basic information and by motivating you to learn on your own. Therefore, the lectures need to be delivered by knowledgeable, enthusiastic and well prepared speakers. Ask the residents if the conferences help to augment what they are learning clinically? Do conferences encourage them to learn more on their own? Are they interesting? Do they have high quality speakers? Conferences should be synergetic to what you are learning from your patients if they are truly an integral part of the curriculum. Do not downplay the need for a well organized conference schedule.

What is the resident to faculty ratio?

While the ideal faculty to resident ratio has not been reported in the medical literature, several Residency Review Committees (RRCs) have requirements in this regard. Obviously this ratio may vary somewhat by specialty, but by no means should this ratio be less than one full-time teacher for each six residents, not counting the program director. Many university residency programs have a 2:1 faculty to resident ratio. It is also important to determine how many are actually active in the teaching process.

Do residents have an opportunity to provide input into the program?

Most candidates are looking for a program where they will be treated less as a student and more as a colleague. In general, this means that a program that values your opinion is more likely to meet your needs. Residents are the recipients of the educational program, therefore, they are the consumers of the training. All educational efforts should be evaluated by those receiving the education. If a residency program's faculty do not understand this concept, it may be wise to look elsewhere for training.

Is the program director an effective leader and devoted to teaching and administrating his or her residency?

Look for longevity and consistency. A red flag for a residency would be the recent loss of a program director and no adequate replacement at the time of interviewing. Have there been multiple program directors in a short period of time?

Ask current residents if the program director is effective in meeting the needs of the residents. Is he or she an effective liaison between the hospital administration and the residents, meet with the residents often and actively solicit the residents opinions? Our experience has been that residents are responsible citizens who know much about what they need in a good education program. Their input and commentary is important.

Is the residency program innovative?
This factor may be the key for your future practice because you can be certain that medicine will change dramatically during your practice lifetime. How does this program adapt to change? Are there innovative programs to assist you in these transitions? For example, the Institute of Medicine has called for a computerized medical record[2]. Is your program teaching computing and medical informatics? If not, why have they not started a program? Look for innovations in health care delivery as well. Is the hospital or university attempting to use alternate health care providers such as physician assistants? The odds are that most physicians will be using medical extenders, whether they are a family practitioner or an ophthalmologist. Programs that do not recognize this fact may be too conservative to help you prepare for your future practice.

What are the strengths and weaknesses of the program?
If you ask several of your interviewers this question, you will have a sense of how they feel about their program. Residents are particularly candid in this regard. If any of the stated weaknesses are particularly important to you it would be wise to discuss them with the program director or his or her designee. It is important to find out how they are being addressed. Remember there are no perfect people and no perfect programs. What is most important is to determine if there is an organized process for continued program improvement. In the end, all strengths and weaknesses need to be rated with your personal criteria for importance before you accept or reject a program based on the answers to these questions.

What is the program's most recent evaluation from the certifying body (RRC) and are deficiencies being addressed?
This is a measure of quality from an unbiased certifying body, so it is important to find out about their most recent site visit. Ask for

a copy of their most recent RRC letter and then discuss their plans to address their deficiencies. Almost every program has some deficiencies. The number and severity are critical measures of the overall quality of the program.

Can the needs of your family be met and are there support systems for residents (such as recreation and mentors, etc.)?
The best way to find out is to ask residents and faculty about basic needs such as time off, day care, availability of housing and employment opportunities for spouses. It is equally important to determine the feeling of group cohesiveness. Do the residents and families get together outside of work? Does the hospital/program plan social events for residents? Do the residents and faculty seem to enjoy being with each other? Ask about annual events and parties for residents. It is a measure of what they think about you. Are they willing to address all of your needs or only your educational needs? Candidates want a program where they will feel part of a group. Residency training will be much more enjoyable if you find a program that meets these criteria.

In the final analysis; the most successful doctors ask themselves, 'How is this particular program going to help me achieve my career goals?' We believe that monetary and geographical considerations are really secondary to this question in the minds of those who regard career development as their ultimate goal.

PREPARING THE APPLICATION MATERIALS
Once you have gone through the process of deciding where to apply your preparation of the actual application materials is of crucial importance because your application is a direct and lasting reflection of your personality. You are attempting to portray the best picture of yourself that you can.

The required application package contains several pieces. The application form itself will be the first piece of information in your file. Behind this will be your curriculum vitae which often is an amplification of information outlined in the application. Last are your letters of recommendation. All programs will require you to have a letter written by the Dean of your medical school in addition to two to three additional letters from medical school professors that you feel can best support your application.

The personal statement

Writing the personal statement is the part of the application package that results in the most difficulty for the student. This often results in procrastination which leads to later submission of the application materials. To avoid this situation, keep in mind what the residency programs look for in these statements. The personal statements are used to separate out those individuals who have little tact, who are relatively illiterate, or are in some way offensive[3]. In general, they are neither looking for literary geniuses nor are they seeking to find only superhumans. They seek individuals with a strong interest in personal and professional growth.

Certainly, there are some personal statements that will stand out simply as a result of the writer's past accomplishments and excellent literary style. A majority of the personal statements, however, are perfectly acceptable based on the fact that they contain the key elements that program directors expect to see from their applicants. The following information outlines these key elements.

What are your reasons for choosing the specialty? This should be considered early in your essay. What was it that drew you to the specialty over the others? Did you have a difficult time choosing between two specialties and if so, what were the reasons behind your decision? It is helpful to use examples from your previous experiences to elucidate these reasons. Touch upon a recent clinical rotation or research experience. Refrain from using lifestyle and income as important factors in your choice. Although they may have been part of your decision-making process, they should not be portrayed as crucial points.

What are your plans for the future? In addition to answering this in your personal statement, you will also encounter it many times in the interview process. It will be helpful, therefore, to think of your answer early in the process. Do you plan to be a community physician or stay in an academic setting? Many of you may not yet know what type of practice you will prefer, but go ahead and answer the question with your present interests in mind. Also, keep in mind the type of programs to which you are applying. If you are applying to mainly academic programs it makes sense to tailor your response appropriately. If you are applying to both academic and community programs, it may be helpful to explain that you are interested in a clinical practice in conjunction with clinical research and teaching. You can make your description more tangible by using the real-life scenario of a physician who you respect and would emulate.

Accomplishments should be used effectively but sparingly. This is a difficult area for the writer because you must, with humility, mention your important strengths and accomplishments without sounding arrogant or haughty. Fight the urge to simply list your honors and awards. There are places in the application and your curriculum vitae for such lists. In the personal statement use specific accomplishments or distinctions to support, for example, why you believe you will be an excellent surgeon. The quality of the accomplishment is more important than listing a number of awards.

No matter what you submit, make it professional. Always type the material and print it on a laser-quality printer. Be meticulous and use proper grammar and spelling (get help if necessary). Keep the length to one page. If shorter, you will not have enough room to say what you need to and if longer, you will lose the reader's interest. Finally, compose your writing in a standard manner. Consider your physician audience who, in general, are conservative individuals.

The curriculum vitae
As your letters of reference are reflections of yourself in others' eyes, your curriculum vitae (or CV) is a picture that you paint of yourself on the laser printer. Although not all applications will specifically require a CV, it is important that you send one along with all of your application packages. By taking the time to put together a neat, concise document that makes note of your accomplishments, the program director will be able to learn about your strengths at a glance and you will have in mind a framework from which to answer questions about yourself in interviews to come. Table 1-1 shows, in order of appearance, the standard requirements for a proper CV[4,5].

Design your CV so that it is neat and easy to read. If you prepare it yourself use a laser printer. If you do not have access to one, have it done professionally. Check and double-check the document for misspellings and poor grammar. Although there is no optimal length it is best to be concise. There are verbose two page CVs and concise five-page summaries. Unless you are widely published, or have years of experiences, attempt to stay within two pages. This will prevent the reader from losing interest.

Table 1-1. Standard requirements for the proper curriculum vitae given in order of appearance

1. Name	7. Research positions/experience
2. Address and telephone number	8. Publications
3. Career objectives	9. Extracurricular activities:
4. Education:	– Hobbies
– High school	– Outside interests
– College	10. Special training, languages
– Medical school	11. Personal data:
5. Honors and awards	– Marital status
6. Work experience	– Children
(in chronological order):	– Citizenship
– Jobs held for a	12. References
significant time	
– Jobs applicable to medicine	
– Military experience	

Be sure to write what you have been doing over the past several years in chronological order. If you have come up to this point in the standard manner, most of your years will be taken up by schooling. However, if you have taken time off or have time gaps in your work or educational history, it is necessary to explain these periods of time. Figure 1-1 is an actual CV submitted in one of the author's application packages. The format may be used with some modification by any residency applicant.

Letters of reference
Along with your other application materials you will be required to have several letters of reference sent in your support. These include a letter from the Dean of your medical school and other letters which you must ask for yourself. Choosing who writes your letters is very important because they portray how these people view your personality and your abilities.

The Dean's letter. The Dean's letter is a standard format letter that is written as a matter of course for everyone graduating from the medical school. Realize that your Dean's letter will not be a letter of recommendation, rather, it is a letter of evaluation[6]. These letters are often very detailed and include most of your educational history with, of course, a more detailed description of your medical school performance. They often directly quote

Figure 1-1. The curriculum vitae submitted in one of the author's application packages

Ravi Reddy
123 Geddes, Apt. 123
Ann Arbor, MI 48104
Phone: (123) 123-1234
SS# 123-12-1234, DOB: 1-2-67

OBJECTIVE:

Specialization in ophthalmology leading to a career in academic medicine with an emphasis on clinical research.

EDUCATION:

Medical School: MD (expected graduation 6/93). University of Michigan, Ann Arbor, MI 1989–present.

Undergraduate: BA in Biology (Honors). Albion College, Albion, MI 1985–88.

High School: Gaylord High School, Gaylord, MI 1981–85.

HONORS AND ACHIEVEMENTS:

Medical School:

Clinical Honors to date: Ophthalmology, General Surgery, Pediatrics, Obstetrics & Gynecology, Dermatology, and Oculoplastic Research.

Clinical High Pass to date: Neurosurgery, Radiology, Neurology and Orthopedic Surgery.

Basic Science Honors: Pharmacology, Pathology, Neural & Behavioral Sciences, Introduction to Clinical Science II & III, and Microbiology.

Basic Science High Pass: Physiology, Genetics, Introduction to Clinical Sciences I & IV.

University of Michigan Medical Research Scholarship, Department of Neurology. Vice President, UM chapter AMA, MSS.

Undergraduate:

Graduated Magna Cum Laude with Honors.
Who's Who Among American College Students.
Dean's List 7/7 semesters.
Member, Omicron Delta Kappa and Mortar Board Honor Societies.
Member, Beta Beta Beta National Biology Honorary.
Varsity tennis.
Vitek Scholarship recipient (Top Junior Biology major).

High School:

Valedictorian, GPA 4.00/4.00 (class of 250 students).
President, Senior Class.
Vice President, National Honor Society.
Who's Who Among American High School Students.
State Champion in Forensic speaking, Radio Broadcasting.
State Finalist, Varsity Debate.

(continued)

RESEARCH EXPERIENCE:

Dr K. M. Spicer, Department of Radiology, Medical University of South Carolina, Charleston, SC (5/88 to 8/88). 'Renal Image Processing: A Study to Assess the Reproducibility of Present and New Techniques.' Senior Honors Thesis published at Albion College, 1988–89.

Dr A. Dilmanian, Department of Medical Physics, Brookhaven National Laboratory, Upton, LI, NY (1/89 to 5/89). Project and acknowledgement in publication entitled: 'A High Resolution SPECT System Based on a Microchannel-Plate Imager.' *IEEE Transactions on Nuclear Science,* 1990; **37**:687.

Dr M. S. Aldrich, Department of Neurology, University of Michigan Medical School (5/90 to 8/90). Project title: 'The Effects of Hypoxemia on REM Sleep.'

PUBLISHED ABSTRACTS:

Aldrich, M. S., Reddy, R. K. 'Effects of hypoxemia on REM rebound during CPAP in obstructive sleep apnea.' *Sleep Research,* 1991; **20**:196.

Aldrich, M. S., Reddy, R. K. 'Clinical follow-up of sleep apnea patients who have had a trial of nasal CPAP.' *Sleep Research,* 1991; **20**:197.

WORK EXPERIENCE:

9/87 to 5/88 & 8/88 to 12/88 Resident Assistant, Albion College, Albion, MI.

5/88 to 8/88 Summer Research Fellowship, Medical University of South Carolina, Charleston, SC.

1/89 to 5/89 Senior Research Fellowship, Brookhaven National Laboratory, Upton, NY.

EXTRACURRICULAR/VOLUNTEER ACTIVITIES:

Medical School:

Nu Sigma Nu Medical Fraternity, Scholarship and Membership Committees.
American Medical Association.
Intramural basketball.

Undergraduate:

Intramural athletics—tennis (doubles champion), basketball, volleyball.
Senior orientation and registration leader, 1988.
Peer tutor, biology.
Delta Tau Delta National Fraternity, 1986–88.

Other interests/hobbies:

Actively enjoy racquetball, cycling, hiking and skiing.

PERSONAL: Single, never married, excellent health.

LETTERS OF REFERENCE: Four letters of reference will be forwarded to the program director's office.

your evaluations from clinical rotations and comment on how you performed relative to your peers. This sometimes includes class rank but, in fact, almost 60% of Dean's letters do not include an actual ranking[6,7].

What can you do to make your Dean's letter as positive as possible? First, it is important to understand the system that is employed by your school. The letter usually goes out from the Dean of Students, but he or she does not necessarily write all of the letters. The letter may be written by a school committee, by an individual faculty member, or by a student advisor. By knowing who will be writing your letter, you may be able to have some input as to what will be included. Very often, the Dean will request that you submit your CV and personal statement. Once the letter is written, it is often possible for you to read the letter and to make changes. It is vital that you take a very personal approach to this process. Submitting your materials to the Dean as early as possible and taking care of the editing expediently will result in a more accurate and timely letter.

Your final responsibility is to submit an accurate list of program names and addresses to which you are applying. It is very helpful to create your own mailing labels on a computer and give them to the Dean's office as this will expedite the mailing of your letters.

Although most programs will wait for the Dean's letter prior to inviting a student to interview, this is not generally true for the early-match specialties (neurology, neurosurgery, ophthalmology, otorhinolaryngology and urology). Several years ago the Council of Deans set November 1 as the date prior to which no letters could be sent[8]. Due to this, and the fact that the early-match specialties must initiate their applicant review process months prior to the regular-match specialties, the Dean's letter is often read after interviews are granted.

Other reference letters. In contrast to the Dean's letter, you have complete control of who writes your letters of reference because it is fully your responsibility to personally ask them to do so. There are several factors to consider in obtaining these letters, the most important being whom to ask.

If the circumstances were perfect, you would choose the most respected, most well-known physician in the specialty to which you are applying. Furthermore, this physician knows you through a working relationship and thinks that you are the best medical student he has ever taught (which he will write in the letter!). Although finding such a reference letter is next to impossible, it is important to get as close to this scenario as possible.

Most schools require three letters in addition to your Dean's letter. Also it is often a requirement that one of these letters is written by the chairman of the department at your school of the specialty to which you are applying. Even if it is not a requirement, it is a good idea to arrange a rotation and speak with them far in advance so that you may obtain a credible letter from him or her. This may be an intimidating thought but your actions and foresight will pay off handsomely in the end, especially in light of the fact that many program directors put more importance on the chairman's letter than they do the Dean's letter[9].

Other excellent reference letters are from clinical professors with whom you have had a significant amount of contact. Preferably, your second letter should also be from a faculty member in your future specialty. Mentors or advisors are often good professionally. Look also to rotations where you were recognized to have done outstanding work. Be careful to choose people from specialties closely related to yours. A letter from a physiatry attending, for example, may not be effective if you are applying for an otorhinolaryngology position. But a letter from a general medical or surgical attending should be helpful for any specialty.

Many students will have done well in basic science courses and look into obtaining a letter from their professors. Avoid this because when applying to clinical specialities it is important to have letters reflecting your clinical acumen. Students often have a background in research. Letters from research faculty can be helpful if the work is somehow related to your field and/or clinical in nature. A good rule to keep in mind is to have the letter from your research faculty serve as your third letter or as your backup letter.

Finally, there are reference letters that will not help your application. These are letters from house staff, friends, relatives, church leaders (pastors and fathers, etc.) or patients. This may seem like common sense but such letters of reference have been submitted in applications for graduate training, such as the National Residency Matching Program (NRMP)[3].

APPLICATIONS: NRMP AND OTHERS

There are a variety of different applications that exist based on the specialty to which you are applying. To limit paperwork a uniform application was created called the *Graduate Medical Education Application* for Residency. In addition to this standard application, a *Central Application Service* has been created for the specialties of neurology, neurosurgery, ophthalmology, and otorhinolaryngology. To get more specific information on how to proceed in the application process in these specialties, write to the specific program address for the materials. Some residency programs, for a variety of reasons, do not accept such standardized applications. They create their own application to make their screening of candidates more efficient. Some residency programs choose to accept either their own or a standard application form. It is advisable that you complete the form that the program provides you. The program director may look upon you more favorably because he sees that you put forth the effort to fill out their form instead of simply submitting a copy of what you have sent to several other programs.

To acquire the applications, you must write to the National Residency Matching Program (NRMP) for an NRMP application packet, which may also be available at your Dean's office. The addresses for the specialty programs are listed in Table 1-2. The first address is to request the American Medical Association's (AMA's) 'green book' which lists all of the programs accredited by the Accreditation Council for Graduate Medical Education (ACGME). In it you will find all the program's addresses and phone numbers listed by specialty and state.

Table 1-2. Useful addresses and numbers for applications into specialty programs

American Medical Association Order Department OP416793, PO Box 109050, Chicago, IL 60610-9050, USA. (Tel: 1-800-621-8335.)	National Residency Matching Program (Directory and Application), 2450 North Street, North-West Washington, DC 20037-1141, USA.
American Urology Association, 6750 West Loop South, Suite 900, Bellaire, TX 77401-4114, USA. (Tel: 713-665-8888. Fax: 713-665-7898.)	Neurology, Neurosurgery, Ophthalmology and Otolaryngology Matching Programs, PO Box 7999, San Francisco, CA 94115, USA. (Fax: 415-923-3945.)

THE INTERVIEW DAY

After the many hours of effort you have put into your application package, you will be rewarded with interviews by the programs who want to meet you. The interview process should not be foreign to you after going through them for college and medical school. Although your previous interviews were crucial in getting into schools, these take on added importance because they are often the most critical factor in getting you into a training program that will determine your life's vocation! Throughout the interview process, preparation and organization will be the keys to your success. The following information outlines important steps to follow.

Gathering data

During the preparation of your application package, continually gather data on the programs you are visiting. This may include a library search to find the research interests of the faculty of a specific department. Also, much insight may be gained from speaking to other students who have interviewed at a program previously. Be active and aggressive!

While gathering this information, you will notice that you will accumulate a significant amount of paper. To deal with this prepare a file for each program that you will be visiting for an interview. In it, place a copy of the application package you sent to them, and all of the information you have gathered on the program (including the information the program sent you). It will be very helpful to go through this file just prior to your interviews (e.g. on the plane or in the hotel room the night before). After you finish your visit and interview, place all communications to and from the program in your file. You will be surprised how important these files will be to you when it comes time to prepare your final match list.

Mock interviews

Prior to the interview, predict and make a list of possible questions that will be asked and answer them on paper first, then verbally prior to your interview. Your answers will be tested when you participate in the mock interview which should be one of the first steps in your preparation for the interview process. Mock interviews are commonly set up by academic institutions for their students. One of the author's (Ravi Reddy) mock interviews was through the career advancement center at the University of Michigan. To set up such an interview, visit the counseling office and do some searching. This author's interview was done by a trained interviewer who knew questions that would be asked by program directors. This experience had real value, because no matter how much I thought about the answers to questions, my real-life interview experience was inevitably different than how I imagined the situation. Be sure to treat the mock interview just as you would a real interview. Wear the same attire, take in the same materials, and have your answers ready.

After the interview, it is crucial to get substantive feedback from your interviews. Additionally, you will also have many thoughts on how it went. Write down exactly what about the interview made you uncomfortable or caused you difficulty. Just imagine, these difficulties would have occurred in your real interviews, but now you have time to correct them prior to the real event. Undoubtedly, this will result in added confidence during the real interview. If you are unable to set up a mock interview it will be helpful to speak to a friend or another student who has successfully gone through the interview process. This will not only give you an idea of the questions asked, but how he or she responded to them and how the interviewer reacted to their answers. They may even be willing to be the mock interviewer.

Your questions for the interviewer
After the interviewer is finished asking you questions, you will be given the chance to ask questions yourself. It is essential for you to have prepared several questions ahead of time to show that you have put some time into thinking about the important considerations of a program.

Write notes on the interview day
Throughout your interview day, make a written note of all of the professors and residents you meet and of anything you liked or disliked about the program. It will be important later that you have all of the names of the faculty members with whom you interviewed (correct spellings, of course) and information you learned about the program during the course of the visit. If you are too busy during the day, make the notes that evening. The longer you wait, the more you will forget to write down and much of the flavor of the day will be lost.

Post-interview communications
Once you have completed your visit and interview you need to write thank you letters to those faculty that took the time to interview you. In addition to the thank you, the letter also serves the purpose of helping the faculty

member remember you. To do this, try to make the letter as personal as possible. You will not be the only applicant writing these letters so use a specific tidbit from your conversation with them.

At some programs you will encounter group interviews where you may not even personally meet all of those in the group. In these instances you may consider writing thank you letters to the chairman and the program director of the department instead of to each and every faculty member in the interview[3].

Everyone is a potential interviewer

One very important practical point. Consider everyone you talk to during your hospital visit as a potential interviewer. Program directors have a close professional relationship with their secretarial staff. An abrupt and demanding demeanor with the program director's office coordinator can hurt your chances while a relaxed and pleasant interaction has the potential to help your interview be a success.

Possible interview questions

All interviewees need to consider the questions that you are likely to encounter during the interview. You must prepare and organize your thought processes and answers to these questions before you can present yourself as confidently and as positively as possible[10,11].

The interview is a time to put formality aside in an attempt to allow the program director to see if there is compatibility between your values and those of the program and institution. The questions are often open ended, without a clear right or wrong answer. Interviewers are looking to see if you have a passion for your work, family and community. At the same time they may be looking for your verbal ability and your capacity to think in a pressured situation.

Why did you choose this specialty? This question may seem obvious to you and you may feel as if you have answered it numerous times in your application package. Nevertheless, this question will probably be asked more than any other. Although there are many ways to approach the questions, look back and define tangible reasons that made an impact on your decision. Did you have an exciting clerkship or a particularly exemplary mentor that was a practitioner in your chosen field? What specifically about the field draws you to it? By addressing these sorts of issues you will have an excellent basis to convince your interviewer.

There are a couple of major pitfalls regarding this question that you must avoid. First, and this applies to all questions; be enthusiastic when giving your answer. It is commonly understood that how you say something is often as important as what you say. Because you will be answering this question so often, your response may get a little dry or stale. Counteract this by conveying your thoughts a little differently each time. We all know that you are excited about entering your specialty, now show it! You may be tempted to prepare to deal with more difficult questions in interview. Avoid this mistake and spend time on your answer just as you would in preparation for the others.

Where do you see yourself in 5 to 10 years? There are two main things that the interviewer is attempting to elicit from you with this question— have you thought about your career and life after your training and is your vision at all plausible? One way to deal with this question is to visualize what kind of practice would be ideal in your mind. Do you see yourself in a rural town with a busy clinical practice or in a large tertiary care center with teaching and research responsibilities? Prior to answering, be sure to think about the type of program that you are visiting. The interviewer will know the training goals of their respective programs. If it is an academic program training research-oriented physicians and you aspire to practice as a community physician, or vice versa, your goals will not match very well.

Another aspect to consider is that a significant number of residents change their career goals during their training. With this in mind, it is probably best not to paint a rigid and specific picture of your future. You may state that you have certain expectations at this point in your life but that you will allow for changes. You will also be asked if you are planning to subspecialize. Deal with this in the same way and keep your flexibility. If you have any interest in subspecialization go ahead and indicate the interest but be careful not to completely rule out other possibilities.

What are your strengths and weaknesses[3,12]? This question may be broken up into two parts or the interviewer may choose to ask you either about your strengths or about your weaknesses. With this in mind, expect any variation and be ready to answer both questions. Your answer will tell the interviewer many things about you. It will become readily apparent whether or not you are tactful, confident, pessimistic or optimistic. Try to avoid the extremes of arrogance and self-defeatism but attempt to keep everything in a positive light. No one likes to listen to a braggart, so try not to hang yourself by being one. One idea is to explain a certain strength through an example. You may illustrate your sensitive nature by the fact that you often make close relations with patients whom you have treated. If you have diverse interests, explain these interests through examples. Above all, be to the point. Verbosity will inevitably either bore the listener or cause you to stumble in your statements[11].

Now for the more difficult flip-side of the questions. The goal is to find weaknesses or flaws that will be acceptable to the interviewers[12]. For example, you may say that you are an intense person when it comes to your work. This trait is often helpful if a person seeks a career in surgery or critical care. Conversely, it may be less helpful if you are a psychiatry resident. In your explanation, believe in what you are saying. The program director's basis for this question is to get a feel for your insight.

Why did you apply to our program? This is a very common question which serves to determine how strong your interest is in that program. If you have taken the time to really look into a program based on the materials you have read and from other students who know the program, coming up with an answer should be no problem. Your rationale may be as simple as geographics, but show the program some respect and add that your interest in the program also stems from the good things you have read and heard about it. As in previous questions, cite specific examples of what you are impressed with (reputation for research, specific projects that you are interested in pursuing, strength of the faculty, etc.).

What if you do not match? This question is probably asked more commonly by the early-match specialties but may be asked by anyone. The keys to answering this question are commitment and preparation. Show that you have considered all the possibilities and that you have plans if you do not match. You must be careful that you do not give up too easily. If you do not match, are you simply going to switch to a specialty that is easier in which to match? Hopefully not! Be committed enough with your decision to take some time to do additional research or rotations to bolster your application package the next time you apply.

Why should we take you over the others[3]? This is a similar question to the 'strengths and weaknesses' question discussed above. This question requires a great deal of tact on your part because it is, once again, an opportunity to hang yourself by rambling on or bragging. Another way to really hurt yourself is to degrade the other applicants in any way. Make it a point to say that the other applicants are also very qualified, otherwise they would not have been asked to interview, but you feel that you have qualities that will help you become an excellent resident.

Some of the qualities that are important to program directors include: the ability to work with others, insight, empathy, devotion to work and family, the desire to distinguish oneself by outstanding patient care, research, writing, or other areas that may be related to medicine. Be sure to clarify these points concisely.

With what subject or rotation did you have the most trouble? There were undoubtedly times in your medical school experience when you had some difficulty which resulted in a poor grade or marginal evaluations. It is best to be straightforward in your explanation. If there were circumstances beyond your control (death in family or illness, etc.), you may, of course, bring these to attention. If, however, it was due simply to lack of effort on your part be careful not to offer excuses. It is a rare student that has a completely unblemished record so deal with it as honestly as possible.

Another way to grapple with this question is to make your difficulty as acceptable as possible. You may say, for example, that you had trouble with the internal medicine board exam because the large amount of time you spent with your patients made it difficult to read as much as you wanted. This tells the interviewer that you were at least very committed to your clinical duties and your final grade did not necessarily reflect your hard work.

Tell me about an interesting patient. The best way to deal with this question is to have prepared for it beforehand. The interviewer can assess many things with this question. You have the opportunity to show what you know and the desire to know, in addition to showing compassion and your ability to interact with patients. You may feel the urge to explain a patient's interesting disease and its pathophysiology, but the question deserves a more far-reaching answer. Did you ever feel helpless or discouraged by the fact that you did not have a cure to offer? Were there quality of life issues? Did you have to deal with the patient's family?

Tell us about a time where you had to work under pressure? The interviewer will obviously prefer a person who works well under pressure. If you explain how you dislike or avoid pressure situations, he or she will be leery about how you can handle a residency situation where there can be significant amounts of stress. Give an example of when you performed well under pressure. Explain how the situation arose and how you reacted (are you usually calm or do you get flustered?). In the end, your goal will have been to convince the interviewer that you are up to the pressure that the residency will place on you.

What type of people do you work the best with?/What people do you have difficulty working with[13]? One of the reasons behind these questions is to determine how you get along and work with other people in general. Residency programs tend to be small, tight-knit groups. For this reason it is very important for the faculty to avoid the difficulties that a disruptive personality can cause. Clearly, people prefer to work with others that are pleasant, helpful and intelligent. The challenge in this question is to explain who you have difficulty working with and how you deal with them. You might have had, for example, an especially demanding and not-so-personable attending or resident while you were a student. You might explain that you took this situation as a challenge and turned it into a positive experience by concentrating on working hard and learning as much as you could from them. It is nice to get along both professionally and socially with your colleagues, but it is important that you can work well with others even if they do not share similar social interests.

What is the most significant thing you have done in the past 5 years? This question provides the interviewer insight into what you find important in your life. Give this question much thought prior to your interview. Some may point to research they have done or to chapters they have written. Others will point to community service projects they enjoyed. I spoke to one student who said that taking care of a sick sibling was the most important thing he had done. While you ponder your answer, keep in mind that the interviewer is looking for a person interested in the process of developing into an excellent physician and humanitarian.

Do you have any hobbies?/What do you do in your spare time? Here the interviewer is trying to assess whether or not you have any interests outside of medicine. Sports are a popular extracurricular activity with many obvious benefits. Although sports are a perfectly acceptable way to spend spare time, many faculty also like to hear of other interest in avenues such as music, drama or literature. For those of you who are married, this is an excellent time to talk about how much you enjoy spending time with your wife or husband and children.

Have you ever been terminated from a job?/Why?/How did it affect you[13]*?* This will not apply to many of you, but those of you who have been terminated need to answer this question thoughtfully. Be straightforward about the situation and spend some time explaining how it affected you and what you did to come back. Maybe your performance was sub-par because you were not stimulated by the job. Having to do work without a future hopefully motivated you to look into your present, more challenging, career path. There is also a sense of failure associated with being 'fired', even from a job that you dislike. It is important to show that you did not wallow in this failure. Rather, it made you re-evaluate your direction and find areas that were more exciting to you.

Tell me about your research. This is a question that should make you shine. There are times, however, when this question can make you look very bad indeed. This occurs when the interviewer asks questions regarding your research that you cannot answer simply because it was several years ago and you did not take the time prior to the interview to review it. Anything in your personal statement or CV is fair game. You might have mentioned, even in passing, something about a research project that you were involved in during your first year of college. Not reviewing the basic tenets of that project may cause you to look either as if you were uninterested and simply padding your resumé or worse yet, fabricating the project.

Where else have you interviewed? This may not sound like a pertinent question to you but do not be alarmed by it. The interviewer is trying to get a feel for who the competition is. The most important point here is to not say anything derogatory about the other programs thinking that will win you favor where you are interviewing. On the contrary, the faculty will most likely wonder how you will put down their program at the next institution you visit. So simply list the programs and if asked, convey some general pleasantries about the other programs.

What do you think about the changes in health care? At first glance, this question seems impossible because of its enormous scope. The interviewer is doing one of two things here. He or she is either attempting to find out whether or not you have taken an interest in medicine's future or setting the stage to make his or her own views on the subject known.

It is probably best to initially answer such a broad question with some general statements. Because the political climate and issues are changing almost daily, it will be important that you stay abreast of these issues especially around the time that you are interviewing. Although these issues are not making a direct impact on you presently, they are certainly impacting the way that your interviewer is practicing. It may be helpful to speak to practicing physicians to get their perspective on changes that are occurring and to find out what the major practical issues are at the present time.

What aspects of your career do you like the best? Obviously, there are a myriad of possible answers here. Most physicians enjoy the challenges posed to us in terms of the amount of knowledge to learn and assimilate, the difficulties of diagnosis and the ways of treatment. You may also have a unique reason for going into a certain field. You may want to use your training to do voluntary work in lesser developed countries or may be involved in missionary work. In a less practical sense, you may simply enjoy the cerebral aspect of medicine while others may enjoy using their hands for treatment. The bottom line is that your answer should be a personal one and should reflect your thirst for professional growth.

Interesting non-medical questions to ponder. There are a number of questions that interviewers may ask you that you will not expect regardless of how much you prepared. The questions are worded such that the answers will be highly personal. In response to these questions, take a deep breath and give it your best shot! Some examples are:

(1) If you could have dinner with three people from the past, who would they be and why?

(2) If you were stranded on a desert island, what book would you want with you?

(3) What was the last book you read? Do you have a favorite book?

(4) What is your most fond memory? Your least fond memory?

(5) Any ethical dilemma (colleague abusing drugs and your position on euthanasia, etc).

SUMMARY

The residency application and interviewing process offers great challenges for professional growth. The process really represents a mirror image of you for program directors. In the end, your intelligence, honesty and creativity will assist you along the way. If you are successful, you may be the interviewer in the future!

REFERENCES

1. Simmonds, A. C. IV, Robbins, J. M., Brinker, M. R., Rice, J. C. and Kerstein, M. D. (1990). Factors important to students in selecting a residency program. *Acad. Med.*, **65,** 640–3
2. Dick, R. S. and Steen, E. B. (eds). (1991). *The Computer-based Patient Record: An Essential Technology for Health Care.* Institute of Medicine. (Washington, DC: National Academy Press)
3. Iserson, K. V. (1990). *Getting Into a Residency. A Guide for Medical Students.* (Columbia, SC: Camden House)
4. Yate, M. L. (1988). *Resumes that Knock 'em Dead.* (Holbrook, MA: Bob Adams Inc)
5. Beatty, R. H. (1984). *The Resume Kit.* (New York: John Wiley & Sons Inc)
6. Hunt, D. D., MacLaren, C. F. and Carline, J. (1991). Comparing assessments of medical students' potentials as residents made by the residency directors and deans at two schools. *Acad. Med.*, **66,** 340–4
7. Toewe, C. H. and Golay, D. R. (1989). Use of class ranking in deans' letters (brief communication). *Acad. Med.*, **64,** 690–1
8. Wagoner, N. E. and Suriano, J. R. (1992). Recommendations for changing the residency selection process based on a survey of program directors. *Acad. Med.*, **67,** 459–65
9. Wagoner, N. E., Suriano, J. R. and Stoner, J. A. (1986). Factors used by program directors to select residents. *J. Med. Educ.*, **61,** 10–21
10. Edis, M. (1989). The interview 1. Rules of the game. *Nurs. Times*, **85,** 54–5
11. Edis, M. (1989). The interview 2. Games people play. *Nurs. Times*, **85,** 45–57
12. King, N. (1987). *The First Five Minutes: The Successful Opening Moves in Business, Sales and Interviews.* (New York: Prentice Hall Press)
13. Yate, M. J. (1990). *Hiring the Best.* (Holbrook, MA: Bob Adams Inc)

2

Moving and renting

B. S. Jammu

INTRODUCTION

The residency years will bring with them a variety of new experiences such as the landlord–tenant relationship. Your experience as a tenant can be gratifying or frustrating, depending on your knowledge of your rights as a renter. The following chapter will provide information that will assist you in your renting and moving experiences.

YOUR RIGHTS AS A TENANT

A common misperception regarding tenancy is that the landlord has exclusive rights at any time to enter or otherwise change the property during a period of tenancy. The first part of this chapter is designed to alleviate this myth and educate the tenants on their rights. The topics covered to accomplish this goal include legal and illegal clauses found in leases, legal and illegal actions a landlord may take, and tips on expeditious moving.

This chapter does not give legal advice but provides a general overview of the nature of your rights as a tenant. The statements presented in this chapter are based on laws in Michigan, California and New York, and may not apply in other states. Therefore, anyone who has a dispute with their landlord is advised to consider legal counsel.

Definition and types of tenancy

Tenancy occurs *when a landlord or landlady, who is entitled to possession of property, grants an exclusive right of possession to another person called a tenant.* There are two types of tenancy:

(1) *Definite,* where there is a written contract between the landlord and the tenant for a definite period of time such as a month, a year, or longer; and

(2) *Indefinite or 'at will',* which is merely a verbal or oral agreement between the landlord and the tenant. Since there is no written contract, this agreement can be terminated by either party at any time.

Leases

The two common types of leases (or contracts) are therefore oral and written. The main issues with oral leases are the amount of rent and the payment of a security deposit. Although this type of lease may be legally binding, it is so infrequently used that we will not discuss them further.

The majority of leases are written by landlords in an attempt to protect the property owners' investment. However, there are laws that protect the interest of the tenant. The *Consumer Protection Act* (CPA) prohibits 'unfair, unconscionable, or deceptive methods, acts or practices in the conduct of a trade or commerce,'[1] and includes the leasing of real property in the definition of trade or commerce (real property is immovable such as land or buildings). In other words, this Act is designed to prevent the landlord from taking advantage of naive tenants by prohibiting illegal clauses. The CPA may have a different name in some states. The CPA affects written leases in two important areas:

(1) The lease clauses that appear to waive rights that are not subject to waiver; and

(2) The lease clauses claiming the right to attorney fees, eviction without court order and prohibiting children.

Landlords may not use written leases to take advantage of tenants who, because of disability, illiteracy or inability to understand the language of the agreement cannot protect their interests. Anyone who suffers because of deceptive practice may make a claim for the actual damages and may recover reasonable attorney's fees. Violations of the CPA are also violations of the *Truth-in-Renting Act* (TRA)[1], which generally prohibits certain objectionable provisions previously found in written leases, for example, clauses that discriminate and exclude certain persons or waiver of security deposit rights, etc.

Extent of the landlord's rights and liabilities

This section will look at the landlord's interference with peaceful possession; the liability of the landlord for injury to the tenant, and guests on the tenant's property; utility terminations; law-suits to collect rent; tenant's security deposits; rent increases; and lastly, discrimination in housing.

Landlord's interference with peaceful possession. If the landlord and tenant have a dispute which leads to the landlord threatening eviction, the landlord cannot use physical force, remove personal property, terminate utilities or change the locks. This is called self-help eviction[2] and is illegal in most states. However, in some states, self-help evictions are legal. Thus, it is important to check the laws in your state or consult legal counsel. The only grounds for a landlord's entrance to the tenant's apartment without permission is a court order, the need to make 'necessary' and 'temporary' repairs, or when the tenant has abandoned the property. If the landlord does change the locks, the tenant may peacefully regain possession by breaking the locks as long as the landlord is not present and physical confrontation is not threatened. If the tenant is still not able to regain possession, then the tenant may take legal actions against the landlord, call the police department to determine if it has a unit specializing in landlord–tenant or consumer disputes, or write to the landlord reminding him that self-help evictions are illegal (when applicable) and that potential damages are accumulating while the tenant remains out of possession[2].

Liability of landlord for injury on the property. All leases and rental agreements are now deemed by law to include an 'implied warranty of habitability'[3]. This means that whether it is written down or not, and whether the landlord likes it or not, he or she is required to keep the place in a habitable condition at all times. If the tenant or guests of the tenant are injured as a result, the landlord is liable, for instance, if the injuries arose out of the condition of the premises (such as a tenant falling on a broken step, slipping on water from a leaky pipe or falling on an unlighted hallway or stairs) or damages arose out of the criminal acts of another. An example of this would be a situation where there is inadequate security and the apartment is robbed or the tenant is mugged on the property, the tenant can recover their losses from the landlord. In the lease, the landlord cannot waive these liabilities.

Utility terminations. If the landlord is providing the utilities, they can only be terminated temporarily to make repairs. In addition, some cities may have a moratorium against termination of utility or services during the cold season. No utility company is allowed to disconnect service to a residential customer between October 10 and April 15 for failure to pay for such service[1]. If you would like to know if your city is protected with a similar moratorium, contact the Public Service Commission in your state.

Lawsuits to collect rent. The landlord does have the right to collect past due rent from a tenant who has moved out of the property (via a lawsuit). If evicted, however, the tenant is relieved from liability to pay rent unless there is a clause in the lease. If the tenant vacates and the landlord indicates, by word or deed, an agreement to accept the premises, such action constitutes surrender thereby excusing any future payment of rent[1].

Tenant's security deposit. Prior to moving in, the tenant must pay a security deposit in addition to the first month's rent. The security deposit is used to pay for any damages the tenant makes during the course of his or her stay. From personal experience, holes created by nails to hang up pictures is not considered damaging and one is not usually charged. However, this is not a law and so it is wise to inquire about this when renting. In addition to the security deposit, there is a nonrefundable carpet or drapery cleaning fee. However, the carpet fee is not included in the *Landlord–Tenant Relationship Act (AKA Security Deposit Act)*. The *Security Deposit Act* (SDA) determines the amount of the deposit, the use of the deposit and the transmittal of information. The amount of deposit has been limited to 1–1½ month's rent in addition to the first month's rent[1].

The SDA requires the landlord to deposit the money in a regulated financial institution and the name and address of that institution is to be given to the tenant. The landlord may use the money only if a bond is posted in its place, insuring that money will be available for the return of the deposit. From my personal experience, this information is usually provided in the lease.

The SDA also requires the necessary information be transmitted with respect to the location of the parties, the condition of the property upon entry and the condition upon vacation. To protect the tenant from phantom landlords, where tenants only know the identity of the resident caretaker, the landlord is required to provide his or her name and address for receipt of communication within 14 days of the tenant's assuming possession. The landlord is also required to inform the tenant of the tenant's obligation to provide in writing a forwarding address to the landlord within four days after termination of occupancy.

The only items for which the security deposit can be used are utility bills not paid by the tenant, past due rent, and 'actual damages to the rental unit...that are the direct result of conduct not reasonably expected in the normal course of habitation of a dwelling'[1]. It is important to note that the 'actual damages to the rental unit' do *not* include the normal wear and tear of drapes or rug during the course of habitation. A separate carpet fee is assessed for this. However, if the rug has unremovable stains (due to paint or wine, etc.) then money can be taken out of the security deposit.

Rent increases. Generally, there is no limitation upon the amount of rent that a landlord may charge. In some states, they may have rent control in certain communities — this is something you may want to investigate. In the *Michigan Residential Landlord–Tenant Law* (pages 68–71) there are four limitations on the landlord's right to raise rent:

(1) The landlord cannot raise the rent during the term of the lease;

(2) The landlord cannot raise the rent in retaliation to a tenant who exercises any of his or her rights;

(3) The *Michigan Consumer Protection Act* states that a landlord cannot charge a rent 'which is grossly in excess of' rents for similar houses or apartments; and

(4) The landlord is generally prohibited from increasing the amount of rental payments under the *Truth-in-Renting Act.*

Discrimination in housing. Sometimes, a rental agent (and rarely a landlord him- or herself) may tell you that he will not rent to African-Americans, Asian-Americans, Arab-Americans or people with Spanish surnames, etc. This does not happen as often anymore because these people learn that they can be penalized for discrimination.

Today, there are more subtle forms of discrimination. For example, if you phone to see if a place is still available, the landlord may say it has been filled if he hears a foreign accent. If he says it is vacant, then you come to look at it and he sees that you are African-American, Chicano or Indian, etc., he could say it has just been rented or that the advertisement misprinted the rent, which is $765, not $675. There are many variations to this theme. If you believe that you are being discriminated against, the best way to check is to run an experiment. Have someone who would not have trouble with discrimination (for example, a white male with no children) to revisit the place soon after you leave and ask if the same unit is available. If it is available, he should also enquire about the terms. The landlord was probably discriminating against you if the response is better. Make sure that your friend's references, type of job and lifestyle are similar to yours so the landlord cannot later say he took your friend and turned you down because of these differences[3].

Race and color are not the only areas where discrimination is found. The *Elliot–Larson Civil Rights Act* prohibits any form of housing discrimination not only on the basis of race, color, religion and national origin, but also on sex, marital status, age, height and weight[4]. However, it is important to note that since 1981, nine states, the District of Columbia and many cities have prohibited discrimination in rental housing against families and children. The refusal to rent to a tenant with children constitutes age discrimination. Federal law also precludes discrimination, but does not include age as a prohibited criterion. Therefore, it is wise to check this in the state you are renting.

If you feel that discrimination has occurred contact your local state agency on fair employment and housing.

PRACTICAL ASPECTS OF MOVING

Many medical professionals must move from state to state or city to city, which can be a very stressful experience. The following are some tips that will help make the process more tolerable. The following advice is given by Beverly Roman, who has moved more than 15 times in 29 years[5].

Issues which must be settled early

These include whether to live in an apartment, condominium or house, and whether to live in the city or suburbs. Then you must decide when you are going to move. The greatest number of people who relocate do so between May and October — thus, dates and equipment should be reserved as early as possible. This applies to moving with professional movers or moving on your own with rental equipment. If moving with professional movers, contact several moving companies and compare cost estimates, pick-up and delivery procedures, insurance protection plan and services. If time is of the essence, you might want to consult the *Consumer Reports* magazine which has recently rated moving companies[6].

Moving yourself

If you have the time, are short of funds, and have many friends, you might want to consider moving yourself. You can start by acquiring all the boxes needed. The boxes can be attained from convenience stores, grocery stores and liquor stores. The boxes from liquor stores are especially helpful because they are sturdy and have partitions that give added protection for glasses, vases, and small breakable items. Any paper that can serve as wrapping paper should be saved as well. A caveat goes out to those who like to wrap items in newspaper — beware, the ink will rub off! Other items you might want to collect are rope, old blankets, package-sealing tape, marking pens and labels.

Proper organization

This will facilitate the actual moving, unpacking and acclimatization to your new home. When organizing your move, it is important to make lists for address changes, contact service and utility companies, and itemize the necessities to take with you. Some sample items that might be put on the address changes list are: bank, car registration, driver's license, insurance, voter registration, magazines, credit cards, investments, medical school records and registration office, and frequent flier club. Once a core list is made, it can always be added to or deleted. The service and utility companies should be given a forwarding address for any remaining bills. This is to avoid any unpaid invoices or bills that can blemish your credit record. Some examples of other businesses which may require your forwarding address, are: newspaper, gas company, television and cable, trash collector, electric company, local telephone, long-distance telephone and lawn care service.

Whether you move or not, it is always important to make a room-by-room inventory of all your household goods. Any possessions or furniture that are valuable should be documented with photographs. This is especially important for insurance purposes. This inventory list should also be updated as frequently as possible.

Buying or renting?

Deciding whether to live in an apartment or a house can be an additional stressor to the moving process. Buying a home, townhouse or condominium is generally considered a good investment when compared with renting. When renting, the monthly payments are never seen in any shape or form after they are given to the landlord. After purchasing a home, each monthly payment makes owning the house that much closer. You will gain tax compensation as well. However, before buying a home, you should consider your intended length of stay and whether the down payment is affordable.

There are reasons why people prefer renting rather than buying a dwelling. Some rent temporarily to determine if they like their new position or even location. Some people wait to find a house in an area in which they desire to reside; some wait for a house to be built. However, temporary renting might mean that you may need to break a lease for relocation, for instance. It is important to read the lease thoroughly to know what you are responsible for financially.

The city or the suburbs?

Another domain of continual decisions we face is where to live, the city or the suburbs? Factors you might want to consider when making that decision are parking, crime rate, cultural events and commuting distance. If you contact the newspaper in your new location and have some Sunday editions mailed to you, you will become familiar with the area's real estate market, mortgage rates, news, theaters, places of interest, school activities and sporting events. If you call the hospital in advance, they may inform you of residents who are leaving or who need roommates.

How can moving affect you?

Some residents have a choice in their living situation and some do not. Some residents may experience culture shock, especially if they are from another country. Culture shock is the potentially traumatizing feeling which results from the dramatic change of being transplanted from a cozy, secure existence to an unfamiliar one. This could involve obtaining new and unfamiliar responses to old and familiar habits. This shock could manifest itself in feelings ranging from mild apathy to severe anxiety to difficulty sleeping, headaches, stomachaches, impatience and anger.

These feelings are a result of the stress created when struggling to find appropriate ways to react to a situation that was at one time routine and normal. Methods to deal with the shock include making your life in that new area as comfortable as possible. This could be as simple as hanging pictures of family and friends or obtaining house plants. Calling friends from a former place of residence, sharing your experience with others who are going through the same process, or joining an organization to meet new people are other ways to alleviate the stress. One thing that I found particularly beneficial was getting to know the city — learning about its rich history and culture. Whenever I had an opportunity, I would explore the city to recognize its hidden beauty — the marketplace, the arts institute, museums, architecture and people. If the feeling of homesickness does not pass, a trip to your former home may help. It might even make you look at the former area in a new perspective and make you look forward to returning to your new city. When this occurs, you will start to realize that you are over the culture shock.

CONCLUSION

Renting and moving can be a challenging experience. This chapter has attempted to apprise you of your rights as a tenant and to offer options and advice for you to consider when you move. Careful planning and knowledge will make your change of city or state much more tolerable.

REFERENCES

1. Chard, R. and Reed, R. L. (1983). General index. In *Michigan Residential Landlord–Tenant Practices*, pp. 16–63. (Detroit: Michigan Legal Services)
2. The Reagents of the University of California (1986). In *California Residential Landlord–Tenant Practice*, pp. 282–4. (Los Angeles: Continuing Education for the Bar)
3. Moskovitz, M. and Warner, R. (1991). Repairs and maintenance. In *Tenants' Rights*, 11th edn, p. 9. (Berkeley: Nolo Press)
4. Anonymous (1994). Parties to real estate transactions; brokers or salesmen; prohibited practice. In *Michigan Compiled Laws Annotated*, Sec. 37.2502. (Detroit: MI Legal Services)
5. Roman, B. (1991). Getting started. In *Moving Minus Mishaps*, p. 5. (Hellertown: BR Anchor Publishing)
6. The Consumers Union. (1990). Surviving your next move. *Consumer Rep.*, **55**, 527–31

3

Starting a new job

J. C. Sunstrum

*Intern 'A' has just graduated from medical school,
and takes a well-needed vacation. The vacation is arranged
to be completed two days prior to starting ward duties in a new
city. Although Dr 'A' has arranged an apartment, personal matters
such as opening bank accounts, utilities and telephone will be taken
care of later. When Dr 'A' begins ward duties, and then requests
for time to arrange these personal issues during the first week,
this irritates the third year resident. With all the pressures and
fatigue from being on call, Dr 'A' becomes disorganized
by the third week, and has a major argument with
a head nurse.*

*Intern 'B' just graduated from school,
and also takes a vacation. Ten days prior
to starting internship Dr 'B' arrives in the new city,
and has time to arrange for pertinent personal matters.
Some time is also invested in exploring the regional
cultural and recreational opportunities. Dr 'B' demonstrates
good organizational abilities during the first ward assignment,
and is able to co-operate with the rest of the team. When a
confrontation in the emergency room occurred with a
physician, Dr 'B' properly obtained the support
and intervention of the senior resident
on the team.*

INTRODUCTION

Beginning an internship is simultaneously an exhilarating and yet stressful point in a professional career. At long last you have acquired a professional degree, and now proceed through the sometimes arduous years of clinical training. The assumption of increasing professional and personal responsibilities is a major personal challenge. Residency training for physicians has become an apprenticeship unlike that of any other profession, and requires a strong sense of personal direction in order to fully succeed. With each advancing year of physician training, your role changes significantly.

ROLES OF THE FLOOR TEAM

The intern

Acquisition of a medical degree now allows an intern direct responsibility for patient care, although the guidance of senior house staff and attending physicians is almost always readily available. An intern often feels caught between patient responsibilities and meeting the demands of more senior physicians.

Teamwork requires a clear understanding of how individual responsibilities expand with each year of training (Table 3-1). Hopefully, the intern will have been acquainted with the concept of a floor team at medical school. A floor team typically consists of the senior resident, one or two interns, and probably one to four medical students. Ideally, the supervision of the medical students will be the responsibility of the most senior resident on the team. Interns will require considerable supervision, and must devote a large amount of time to patient care.

An intern's ability to contribute to smooth team operation is enhanced by a willingness to assume responsibilities, combined with meticulous attention to a large number of patient care details. Listing the patients' data on index cards is a valuable technique for organizing priorities (see Fig 3-1).

A most helpful tool, regardless of the type of training program, is a physician's notebook. This should be loose leaf and fit in your white coat's pocket. (A possible alternative could be one of the electronic notebooks, such as the Hewlett Packard 100 LX Palm top computer.) Concise summaries of key lectures, principles, dosage formulas and phone numbers, etc., can all be accessed rapidly. These also provide valuable study notes for later in your training[1].

Table 3-1. Roles during each stage or year of residency training

Year	Responsibilities	Key role
Internship	Initial patient evaluation Routine patient care decisions Organize patients' care	Apprentice Junior teacher
Junior resident	Supervise interns and students Approve diagnosis and management Demonstrate ability to work with other personnel	Team supervisor Teaching role expected Troubleshooter for minor conflicts Key contact person for attending physician
Senior resident	Competent team supervision Able to handle complex patients	Senior advisor for junior residents Conflict resolution of more significant issues Competent team teacher
Attending physician	Assures team can handle essential concepts of medicine Stimulates reading on core materials Reviews charts and orders for completeness	Teacher Mentor Handle major conflicts

The first few months of the internship is the most stressful period in residency training[2]. Confidence in decision-making may be weak, and you often feel constantly pressured from all sides. Working hours and the nature of the duties performed remain controversial areas for training programs. There is no question, however, that long working hours have a significant impact on an intern's personal and family life[3]. In fact, it has been stated that the bleakest times of residency occur during the first year of training, usually on the intensive care rotations[4]. Many programs have set limits on duration of on-call time, and eliminated certain trivial or 'scut' duties (i.e. transport of lab specimens, services on non-teaching patients and other non-educational tasks). 'Scut' is a somewhat noxious and debatable term; certainly many practicing physicians perform similar tasks

```
Name: _____
(or addressograph stamp)

Key problems:
1.
2.
3.
4.

Labs:              Hgb          WBC Platelets
Na      K          CO₂          Cl
BUN                Creatinine
Others

CXR:
Other X-rays:
ECG:

Meds:
1.
2.
3.
4.
```

Figure 3-1. A patient data card. WBC, white blood cells; Hgb, hemoglobin; BUN, blood urea nitrogen; CXR, chest X-ray; ECG, electrocardiogram; Meds, medications

in their daily duties. However, a physician in training is entitled to air concerns if such tasks interfere with their education[5]. In addition, careful written documentation of time spent performing tasks not pertinent to educational objectives provides a powerful incentive for programs to institute effective changes[6]. For example, one study surveyed internal medicine interns on call, and documented 21 beeps per 30 hours. An average of only 2.5 hours of sleep (with two interruptions) was reported, with only 4 minutes of reading time. This survey found attending physicians averaged only 12 minutes of bedside interaction with patients, and resulted in a major re-evaluation of the structure of teaching rounds and night call[6].

The junior resident
The progression from internship to junior resident signals the greatest increase in personal patient responsibility. You will now report directly to

the attending physician, with senior residents available for advice or consultations on questions of major concern. This change in roles will place you in charge of maintaining effective communication with the attending physician, and make you primarily responsible for the operation of the ward team. The junior resident is also expected to teach and supervise medical students on the team.

You must now also be able to provide adequate supervision and teaching to the new interns, a role that many people have difficulty performing. Supervision of another professional in training requires a careful balance of inquiry and trust. Certainly in the first months of supervising a more junior physician, it is appropriate to ask for detailed information to ensure that the intern has indeed performed the necessary work. As the year proceeds, the junior resident can allow the interns to operate more independently as expertise develops.

The senior resident

Individual programs vary in their view of the function of the senior resident. Usually at this stage, a senior physician in training will directly supervise a ward team, acting with experience, and being available to the team at all times. Teaching becomes a prominent responsibility during this period, and it is a challenge to address the educational needs for all levels of the team. It is at this stage of your career that medical knowledge is at its maximum. The art of stimulating discussion on ward rounds is essential, and it is important to first question the most junior members of the team. This will establish a certain educational hierarchy, and helps avoid the embarrassing situation of a junior medical student providing an answer which a senior resident does not know.

The attending physician

Final responsibility for the team rests with the attending physician, who should be relied on to handle the most difficult patient issues or other conflicts which arise. Certainly, he or she must be involved when the team encounters a patient care crisis, or major interpersonal conflict. The attending physician must balance a willingness to allow latitude in judgment, and yet be capable of stepping in when assistance is necessary. His or her clinical experience is an inestimable resource to draw upon, and hopefully the team's up-to-date medical knowledge will enrich the team experience for all involved.

Table 3-2. Principles of conflict resolution

---

(1) A private discussion with the party involved is best, before asking others to intervene. Use a conciliatory approach to avoid emotions taking priority over facts

(2) Seek the assistance of your senior resident, chief resident or attending physician if no satisfactory response is obtained

(3) Document problems to strengthen your case. Facts and numbers carry weight

(4) Program director's involvement is always available if you are not able to get the conflict resolved

---

PERSONAL CONFLICTS DURING TRAINING

Establishing a capacity to resolve the conflicts which inevitably arise on the wards is a major challenge during your training period. Patient management conflicts, whether with nursing staff or attending physicians, are best left to the more senior resident on the team. Conflicts with members of the team should be handled *early*, since procrastination will only aggravate frustrations. Private discussions are vastly superior to discussing a contentious matter in front of others, and under no circumstances should conflicts be raised in front of patients or their families. See Table 3-2, which lists the principles of conflict resolution.

Often interns feel powerless or too unimportant when difficulties arise. House staff must feel empowered to enact changes within the institution, and residency training is an important time to learn these skills. A few of the common complaints of house officers working on ward teams are now discussed.

'My team always seems to carry more patients than other teams'

This can occur, but it may be necessary to evaluate the team's efficiency in managing the patients. If documentation supports a significantly heavier load, then the chief resident is best equipped to handle the situation.

'The nurses are often questioning my decisions'

Nurses are entitled and obligated to question any physician's decision if this is necessary. It is often a moment to learn from other health care personnel, who have years of clinical experience to draw upon. On the other hand, this may be a chance for you to educate other personnel and demonstrate your expertise.

TIME MANAGEMENT

A resident is constantly faced with multiple and often simultaneous demands for information and decisions. It is therefore necessary to prioritize, but this can be difficult for a variety of reasons. Residents often do not have their own individual office, although some programs do at least offer a study carrel or desk. The advent of the modern pager or beeper can make it nearly impossible to avoid interruptions on your time. Nevertheless, the ability to handle requests for your attention will be a major determinant of how you effectively function as a physician, manager and teacher.

There are several philosophical schools of time management principles, and the applicability of each depends on your individual approach and preference. Some management consultants advise professionals to adhere to carefully designed schedules, to avoid interruptions, and suggest multiple categories of priorities[7]. For example, an expert in this field suggests four quadrants of time management:

(1) Urgent/important;

(2) Not urgent/important;

(3) Urgent/not important; and

(4) Not urgent/not important[8].

(See Chapter 4 on Time Management.) An alternative, and more fluid, approach has been recently suggested following analyses of successful senior executives. Rather than rigid control of the day, handling brief unscheduled conversations promptly is now recognized as essential to getting things done quickly and efficiently[8-10] (see Table 3-3).

This strategy is somewhat analogous to the major changes introduced recently in the automobile manufacturing industry in the United States. Rather than maintain expansive and expensive inventories of parts and components, with major record keeping functions, a 'just-in-time' system of delivering parts to the factories eliminates enormous overhead.

Table 3-3. Tips for handling time

(1) Avoid over structuring the day	(4) Think on your feet
(2) Answer pagers promptly	(5) Read up on a problem as soon as possible
(3) Do not postpone decisions	

Although slightly vulnerable to temporary interruptions, this tactic has significantly reduced the costs and time involved in production schedules.

Timely handling of such intrusions on your current activity is essential when managing patients' care. Although each individual has his or her own style, a physician's capacity to care for patients depends heavily on close personal contact. While you do not wish to abruptly cut off a patient interview at a critical point, it is possible to courteously break away at a transition part of the interview. Your ability to promptly respond to calls and pages will enhance your reputation among colleagues and other health care professionals. It is much better to handle the issue directly, rather than try to recontact the caller at a later time in the day or week. In fact, allowing interruptions actually saves time in many circumstances, avoiding the delay and frustrations of postponing decisions[11].

Similarly, when actively involved in managing a patient's case, it is important to be willing to quickly review the medical textbooks or current literature. This is a key opportunity for considerable learning to occur, and the information gleaned is often directly valuable to assisting the care of the patient. This is also a successful strategy for passing board examinations.

COVERING OTHER RESIDENT PHYSICIANS
Working with other busy professionals in training often requires you to 'cover' someone else's duties. For example, on nights and weekends your patients are being followed by the team on call. Vacations, sick and personal days off are other examples where you must clearly delineate who and how your patients are to be covered (see Table 3-4). This is critical not only for your relationships with peers, but particularly for appropriate patient care.

Table 3-4. Do's and don'ts when covering for other physicians

Do

(1) Be sure to identify the patients most likely to be unstable

(2) List all the laboratory tests and X-rays which needed to be checked

(3) Remember to acknowledge your covering teams from time to time

(4) Keep your problem list up to date, to assist other physicians evaluating your patient for the first time

Do not

(1) Neglect to properly determine resuscitation status (i.e. no code) for terminally ill patients

(2) Leave very unstable patients until the on-call physician has a chance to acquaint him- or herself

PERSONAL TIME OFF AND CONFERENCES

Most teams now sign out to the on-call team just prior to leaving the hospital for the day. This alerts the new team to any problems anticipated for the next several hours. Reports should be very concise and practical, since the on-call team will be receiving reports from several teams.

Programs have individual policies for vacation and personal time off, but vacation time will need to be arranged well in advance with your program director in writing (see the checklist in Table 3-5). Hospital operators should be informed of your days off, and told which resident physician will handle your phone calls. These arrangements are critical to avoid hard feelings with both your colleagues and patients. You and your peers will always appreciate the thoughtfulness of prior notification of absences.

Table 3-5. Checklist for vacations and personal days

(1) Notify the program director in writing of your planned time off

(2) Arrange for another resident physician to cover your clinic patients

(3) Notify the hospital telephone operator of your plans and coverage

(4) Leave a forwarding telephone number in case you need to be contacted

When you need to leave on short notice when, for instance, a family emergency arises, these arrangements need to be taken care of despite the emotional overlay of the situation. Your chief resident is available to assist you if complete arrangements cannot be made.

MOONLIGHTING

Few topics stir such controversy as that of moonlighting during your residency training[12,13]. Some claim there are no data indicating that moonlighting is 'dangerous,' and serves an important economic benefit. These proponents feel it is not the business of training programs to scrutinize the activities of house staff outside working time. Certainly, the legal authority of programs over such extracurricular activities is extremely limited. However, opponents of liberal moonlighting activities believe that it detracts from your educational goals, and may exacerbate the malpractice liability of the institutions employing moonlighters who are in training.

Many programs now offer 'in-house' approved moonlighting opportunities, which offers the potential of meeting the above concerns. Nevertheless, any individual who is experiencing difficulties or problems in progressing through clinical training or who has had previous academic problems with standardized examinations should *not* be involved in moonlighting.

SUMMARY

To be a successful physician you must have the knowledge of biomedical science as well as the skills in management. This chapter has provided the basic medical management concepts by outlining the roles of members of a ward team and presenting strategies to manage yourself and others more effectively.

REFERENCES

1. Harrison, M. R. and Adzick, N. S. (1990). Advice to a resident: a surgeon's notebook. *J. Pediatr. Surg.*, **25,** 379–80
2. McCue, J. D. (1985). The distress of internship: causes and prevention. *N. Engl. J. Med.*, **312,** 449
3. McCall, T. B. (1988). The impact of long working hours on resident physicians. *N. Engl. J. Med.*, **318,** 775–8
4. Schwartz, A. J., Black, E. R., Goldstein, M. G. *et al.* (1987). Levels and causes of stress among residents. *J. Med. Educ.*, **62,** 744–53

5. Hayward, R. S., Rockwood, K., Sheehan, G. J. and Bass, E. B. (1991). A phenomenonology of scut. *Ann. Intern. Med.,* **115,** 372–6

6. Nerenz, D., Rosman, H., Newcomb, C. *et al.* (1990). The on-call experience of interns in internal medicine. *Arch. Intern. Med.,* **150,** 2294–7

7. Applebaum, S. H. and Rohrs, W. F. (1981). *Time Management for Health Care Professionals.* (Rockville, MD: Aspen Publications)

8. Winston, S. (1983). *The Organized Executive: A Program for Productivity.* (New York: Norton Inc.)

9. Mintzberg, H. (1973). *The Nature of Managerial Work.* (New York: Harper and Row)

10. Blanchard, K. and Johnson, S. (1986). *The One Minute Manager.* (Random House)

11. Deutschman, A. (1992). The CEO's secret of managing time. *Fortune,* **127,** 135–46

12. Factor, R. M. (1991). Moonlighting: what residents do in their free time is their decision. *Hosp. Community Psychiatry,* **42,** 739–42

13. Keill, S. L. (1991). Moonlighting: why training programs should monitor residents' activities. *Hosp. Community Psychiatry,* **42,** 735–8

4

Time management

M. H. Yurkanin, L. D. Victor and D. D. Hendee

INTRODUCTION

Everyone has demands on their time. How you spend and save your time will define your character and determine your personal and professional success. It is commonly thought that house officers are overworked and have little time left over for their personal lives, contributing to life and job dissatisfaction. This chapter will offer you tips on how to manage your time so that you have additional time for other enriching pursuits that are important to your future happiness.

Inefficient time use

Although most of the time management literature is centered in the business arena, there have been some revealing studies showing the inefficiencies of house officers. Lurie *et al.*[1] found that during a 24-hour call only 87–175 minutes was spent on direct patient evaluation. Most of their time was used doing unsophisticated procedures, such as starting intravenous lines or drawing blood specimens, which could be done by non-physicians. If the house officer's time could be spent more efficiently, there would be more time for direct patient contact or educational pursuits such as reading journals or performing research.

Pareto's principle and time wasters

Many people use their time inefficiently. Early in this century an important idea was formulated called Pareto's 80/20 principle, which states that 80% of time is spent to do 20% of work. This means that time is used so inefficiently that often three to four times the amount needed is used to get the job done. This is because of time wasters: ill-defined goals, priorities and deadlines associated with poor delegation of responsibility and procrastination. Elimination of these time wasters will allow you to accomplish more work in less time. Your goal should be to invert Pareto's principle; that is, to spend 20% of the time to do 80% of the work! The principles of how to accomplish more in less time form the basis of time management.

THE PRINCIPLES OF TIME MANAGEMENT

Set goals
Busy and successful people pursue many personal and professional goals. Knowing what the goal is before starting your task will direct your energies and save time. The following are a few tips on how to set goals.

Short- and long-term goals. First, divide goals into those that are short- and long-term.[2] Although long-term goals alone sometimes make it difficult to see the end product and short-term goals may have an obscure end point, both long-term and short-term goal setting will allow you to define a value and a direction. An example of a long-term goal was to have this chapter finished by the editor's deadline. The short-term goals were to write rough drafts and to edit. Even shorter goals were determined by each author when they decided how many pages to write or areas to research. Short-term goals can frequently be broken down into daily goal setting and planning. Remember to leave room for error, because often there are unforeseen circumstances that can cause delay.

Write goals down and update. Write the goals down and update often as circumstances warrant. Writing goals down and commenting on their progress helps to keep you focused in the right direction.

Set priorities
An important skill in time management is the ability to set priorities. Priority setting begins by putting the first things first[3]. Do the important things first and allow them more time. This may come at the expense of urgent, but unimportant things. Many people want to handle the urgent problem over the important project (e.g. a telephone page from a friend over studying for a board examination); the perception is that talking to

a friend is more pleasurable than studying. This may be true in the short-term, but idle phone conversations will not help you pass tests. Ultimately, which is more pleasurable?

Four quadrant method. The four quadrant method to setting priorities is an effective way to decide what is important vs. what is not important, and what is urgent vs. what is not urgent (Figure 4.1)[2,3].

I. URGENT AND IMPORTANT	II. NOT URGENT, BUT IMPORTANT
Crises **Pressing problems** **Deadline driven projects** *(i.e. cardiac arrests, emergency floor problems, book chapters and family responsibilities)*	**Preparation** **Crisis prevention** **Goals clarification** **Planning** *(i.e. board certification, research projects, continuing medical education, and health and fitness activity)*
III. URGENT, BUT NOT IMPORTANT	IV. NOT URGENT AND NOT IMPORTANT
Interruptions *(i.e. visiting friends and relatives, interruptions to gossip, drug representatives, some pages and most telephone calls)*	**Busy work** *(i.e. moonlighting, buying expensive clothes, buying expensive cars, watching television, pleasure reading, gourmet cooking and excessive sporting activity)*

Figure 4-1. The four quadrant method of setting priorities

Quadrant I activities are easy to recognize (i.e. cardiopulmonary arrests, emergent medical ward problems, book chapters with a deadline and critical family problems). The difficulty arises because these activities require an immediate reaction that may lead to inefficiency, procrastination of more important projects or, on occasion, a poor decision. This is not a totally unavoidable quadrant, therefore it is important to prepare for any of the uncontrollable time spent there (e.g. know the advanced cardiac life support guidelines), prepare for common floor problems, set goals for project deadlines and call your baby-sitter early.

The above recommendations for staying out of quadrant I are all examples of activities in quadrant. II. Quadrant II is the most important quadrant. If quadrant II prevention of crises is neglected, quadrant I crises will cause disruption. Therefore, plan carefully to avoid unnecessary time in the first quadrant. An example would be, if I neglect planning for writing this chapter (quadrant II) by spending all my free time watching football (quadrant IV), I will miss my deadline and be in a crisis (quadrant I). Too much time in quadrant I has the tendency to cause stomachaches, poor sleep and marital discord. More time in quadrant II helps alleviate stress, increase your standard of living and enhance life satisfaction.

Quadrants III and IV contain behaviors that cause trouble. It is often difficult to determine what is urgent, but not important. For example, quadrant III problems include visiting friends. In addition, many telephone pages and calls from solicitors fall into this category. The inexperienced worker gives these activities much more time than they deserve. This quadrant must be controlled to make the four quadrants method more effective. An example would be, if I spend too much time with a drug representative (quadrant III), I will not get reading done to prepare for floor problems (quadrant II) and when I get a page on a patient in new onset atrial fibrillation with unstable vital signs (quadrant I), I will struggle to handle the crisis.

Quadrant IV activities cause the most trouble. They are easy to define but difficult for the unwary and unmotivated to ignore. The pleasant activities (i.e. sports and pleasure reading, etc.) are difficult to avoid. Though these activities serve an important function to emotional well-being, they can often be delayed to spend more time on more important activities. An example would be, if I allowed my friends to drop by (quadrant III) and disrupt my studies for my next set of board exams (quadrant II), by convincing me to go mountain biking (quadrant IV), I may do poorly on board exams, putting me in to a crisis (quadrant I).

Pursuing unrealistic personal values as a resident also can be counter-productive. The resident that has the disorder that we call 'elegantitis' (the desire to become elegant by buying expensive clothes, cars and homes) will be seduced into moonlighting and reducing time on pursuing research projects or studying for board examinations. The resident may have a Corvette but risks failing his or her boards. Elegantitis can be a very serious and destructive character disorder as its presence is a common cause of professional and personal failure among residents.

The above is an example of how the four quadrant method is to be used. It is obvious that quadrant II is where the most time and effort should be spent. Learn to be proactive, by being prepared, as in quadrant II, rather than reactive, as in quadrant I. The activities in quadrant II are the most important to your personal success. Much of the time spent writing this chapter was spent in quadrant II, 'not urgent but important.'

Delegate responsibility

Most physicians are independent people who have a difficult time delegating work. Usually, it is the fear that only they can do the task correctly. Delegating responsibility with the confidence that you can handle any problems created by your subordinates is the sign of an effective manager and physican. Remember, in order to delegate, you have to be able to do the job as well or better than the person to whom you are giving the job. Delegation involves several skills[4], which are now discussed.

Organization. First, organize tasks and decide which are best given to others and those that should be performed by yourself. In the study by Lurie *et al.*[1], house officers were often spending time drawing blood and starting intravenous catheters, etc., which could be delegated to ancillary staff. Choose the best person for the job. Using a nurse to administer medications and laboratory personnel to draw blood is the most efficient use of each person's skills and abilities. Save the most difficult tasks for yourself.

Communication. Learn to communicate effectively. Seek first to understand then to be understood[4]. If you listen carefully to those speaking to you, they will be more likely to listen to your point of view. Your point of view should be clear in your mind, as it is important to know what you want done before you give instructions so that the listener will understand. Then speak assertively, not aggressively, when giving instructions.

Delegating does not end with telling someone to do a job. It is also important to know that the resources are available to the person doing the job so that it can be done correctly. Also, you must follow up with the progress of the job, giving guidance where it is needed and credit where it is due.

A good example of the communication and delegation is the following scenario. A patient with a right-sided pneumonia needs a central venous catheter. It is the middle of the year and the intern is familiar with the procedure. If the senior resident would like to delegate this responsibility to the intern, he or she should convey to the junior house officer that the right internal jugular would be the preferred route as the potential for a catastrophic pneumothorax is less on the side where the major disease is located. In the unlikely event that there is an iatrogenic pneumothorax, there is less chance of life-threatening hypoxemia if the bad lung on the right collapses than the good lung on the left. Moreover, in this more risky situation, the senior resident must be physically present during the actual procedure. Efficient use of time would be to have the junior resident set up for the procedure and then call the more senior resident at the time of the initial venipuncture. Communication, delegation and supervision are imperative in this situation. Both the senior resident and the junior resident are making an efficient use of their time.

DICTATION

Writing is an area of great concern for residents and students. It is very time-consuming to write histories, physicals and procedure notes. Documentation methods other than handwriting are more efficient. Consider the following: most people write in longhand at about 15 words per minute, type at 20–60 words per minute and dictate at 65–95 words per minute[5]. Dictation saves time. Once you get over the initial awkwardness of dictating, you will not want to return to the prehistoric pen and paper approach.

GETTING STARTED

Daily and weekly 'to do' lists are helpful. Make a list and label the activities by priority and follow this as closely as possible, this will help you get the important things done and give you a sense of accomplishment when you take things off your list.

A way to keep everything organized is to use a handheld electronic organizer[6]. These are designed to be a convenient and easy way to carry an appointment book, telephone directory and notepad, etc. They offer an array of features that help people manage their business and personal affairs more effectively.

MANAGE INTERRUPTIONS

Health care professionals are often the biggest culprits in mismanaging their time[7]. They are especially poor at handling interruptions. Generally, they allow others to cause interruptions in their work. These interlopers may include nurses, ancillary staff, superiors and friends. Health care professions should review the four quadrants discussed earlier in the chapter and decide the quadrant in which each interruption occurs, allocating the appropriate amount of time each interruption warrants.

AVOID PROCRASTINATION

Our own misbehavior usually prevents us from reaching our desired goals and objectives. A common maladaptive behavior is procrastination[8], which in the minds of many is a primary reason for professional failure. Regardless of the excuses and behaviors for procrastination, the results often lead to feelings of anxiety, frustration and loss of self-esteem.

Procrastination behaviors can be overcome. They can be modified by first understanding when, where and why we procrastinate. It is helpful to identify the types of situations that prompt procrastination at work, in your personal relationships and in your financial affairs. The four main reasons for procrastination are listed below.

Fear of failure

There are often underlying psychological reasons why we procrastinate. One reason could be the fear of failure, which is probably the most common and least rational cause for procrastination. The key point to keep in mind is that failure is rarely fatal. Moreover, it is through failure that we learn to succeed the next time. How many different compounds did Thomas Edison try before he finally developed the incandescent lamp? Hundreds!

One technique for overcoming fear of failure is to break large projects into smaller tasks and schedule time to complete the component parts of the project. Successful completion of smaller projects can give confidence to deal with procrastination behaviors on the larger projects.

Perfection paralysis

Another major reason for procrastination is that we expect to achieve perfection in everything we do. Perfection is not an option but an obstacle in life. There are three basic questions to ask yourself when faced with the perfection paralysis phenomenon:

(1) What does perfection really mean?;

(2) How much will it cost in terms of time, energy and money to achieve perfection?; and

(3) Is it really worth the effort?

The more realistic goal in most endeavors is to do the best you can with what you have. If you are a country physician with no hospital facilities nearby, your care of a ruptured aortic aneurysm will be considerably different than if you are working in a trauma center of a large city hospital. In either case you will have to devote considerable time and effort to save the patient, but your self-esteem cannot always ride on the outcome, which may be fatal in either case. The process of your effort is what is important. You should strive always to be able to say that "I have done my best", and when the project is over be able honestly to ask yourself, "How could I have done it better?" The perfect outcome becomes less important than the process you took to get there.

Fear of success

There is a fair amount of literature today about women in particular who fear that a successful career can only be achieved at the expense of a family life. For example, women sometimes feel that, if they earn a lot of money, their husband will feel threatened. It is not unusual for some people to sabotage their own success through procrastination. The primary way to overcome the fear of success is to get used to success and feel good about it. Have a sense of purpose or mission in your life. A sense of purpose needs to be perceived as more important than the fear of success.

Lack of self-discipline

Successful people discipline themselves to do the important and difficult tasks first. Although the final result of your efforts is often reward enough to continue working, smaller rewards along the way will often encourage you to work harder.

The reward system is yet another technique for dealing with procrastination. The key is to find something you want more than the task you have been putting off and reward yourself with it. For example, after you have completed a task associated with your research project, reward yourself with a cup of coffee, or something you enjoy. This idea can be taken a step further by incorporating rituals to the things you have been putting off. Having your favorite tea nearby every time you work on your research project could be incorporated as a ritual. In addition, attaching a sense of urgency to a vital goal may make it difficult to put it off until tomorrow[9].

While it may be difficult to change procrastination behaviors and perhaps even more difficult to change old habits, it is clearly more enjoyable to accomplish the things that you want to do. Once you overcome procrastination, you will feel better about yourself and lead a happier, healthier and productive life.

CONCLUSIONS

Time management is how effectively time is spent. Many successful people manage their time very well without ever knowing the principles set forth in this chapter. Most need some guidance. Setting goals and priorities should be done hourly, daily and weekly. Delegating tasks will give you more precious time. Avoidance of procrastination will help get the job done sooner. Finally, consider the four quadrants of time management, focusing your efforts in quadrant II — 'non-urgent, but important.' Remember, it is not time we are trying to manage, but ourselves.

REFERENCES

1. Lurie, N., Rank, B., Parenti, C., Woolley, T. and Snoke, W. (1989). How do house officers spend their nights? A time study of internal medicine house staff on call. *N. Engl. J. Med.*, **320**, 1673–7
2. D'Alton, L. (1991). Stretch your day. Effective time management can add time to your day. *Manager's Mag.*, **66**, 21–3
3. Covey, S. R. (1989). The 7 habits of highly effective people. Simon and Schuster Audio Division, Simon and Schuster Inc, New York. (Audio tape)
4. Buhler, P. (1992). How to work smarter — more than time management. *Supervision*, **26**, 12–13

5. Smeltzer, L. and Gilsdorf, J. (1990). How to use your time efficiently when writing. *Business Horizons,* **33,** 61–4
6. Alvich-LoPinto, M. (1991). Handheld electronic organizers make juggling tasks a breeze. *Today's Office,* **25,** 58–9
7. Mackenzie, A. (1991). Why time management doesn't always work. *Life Assoc. News,* **86,** 99–103
8. Cox, J. and Read, R. (1989). Putting it off 'til later — procrastination: causes and corrections. *Baylor Bus. Rev.,* **7,** 10–15
9. Hobbs, C. (1992). Creative procrastination. *Exec. Excellence,* **9,** 17–18

5

Taking a history the easy way: the health history questionnaire

T. R. Child and L. D. Victor

INTRODUCTION

Increasing documentation is required by all health care practitioners in order to assist the 65 or so separate individuals and agencies accessing the medical record[1]. Central to this documentation is the physician's history and physical examination. Physicians frequently elicit inadequate histories, record data haphazardly, and provide patient and hospital records with incomplete data[2]. This part of the data base is often abbreviated because of inconsistent standards, difficulty obtaining information from patients and families, and a lack of enthusiasm on the part of physicians. Some authors are asking for a more routine and standardized method of data collection[3].

ROUTINE DATA COLLECTION

Why is it avoided by physicians?

Our experience has been that routine data collection is often avoided by physicians because there is little incentive to undertake it. An extended data base is not necessary for managing the patient's immediate problem and the physician is not compensated for the inordinate amount of time required to collect the information. In addition, it is often tedious and boring to ask routine questions. Histories performed as they are taught in medical school may require 1–2 hours to complete[2]. House officers with multiple admissions often attempt to short-cut the history taking process which may result in less than optimal patient care. Adding to the inefficiency of data collection is inexperience. House officers in training may not ask the right questions as shown in one study evaluating the accuracy of junior clinicians in diagnosing appendicitis[4]. Experienced physicians, because of their increased knowledge, often recall more information for the medical record than younger, inexperienced physicians[5]. Personal attitudes toward history taking may also be of some significance. Experienced physicians tend to concentrate on the patient's condition at the time of examination, while younger colleagues spend time extrapolating more details[6].

Patients and data acquisition
Patients may be reluctant to give the time and attention necessary to retrieve a detailed history. They may be frightened or embarrassed and give false or incomplete information. Unless given the opportunity to reflect and consult with other family members, they may be unaware of or have forgotten past illnesses. Patients often write material that they refuse or hesitate to relate verbally[2].

Documenting data
Written documentation on the patient record is another time-consuming chore. It is not unusual to see a decay in the legibility and content of chart documentation as resident work-load increases. Dictating the history and physical part of the medical record would save the physician valuable time and increase chart legibility.

At the end of this chapter is a standard self- or family-administered health history form adapted from one used to obtain a subspecialty history[7]. This health history questionnaire may be used in conjuction with a dictation macro* in order to assist the house offices in collecting data and dictating a standardized history in an efficient fashion.

THE HEALTH HISTORY QUESTIONNAIRE

Self-administered questionnaires
The earliest, standardized, self-administered questionnaire was the Cornell Medical Index[8], which showed that forms could be easily

---

*Macro is a computer term meaning a file containing a series of keystrokes. In this case the keystrokes are the abbreviated headings contained in a standard history and physical examination.

completed by patients. They were particularly helpful in collecting social and psychological data. Other studies showed considerable time savings and using questionnaires allowed staff to spend more time on patient and teaching activities[9]. None of the questionnaires in any of the studies obviated the need for a thorough history of present illness, but they consistently did obtain more useful information. A self-administered history does not replace the physician's interview; with a clinician's assessment of a patient's problems, it complements the interview, physical exam and laboratory testing, providing a more detailed picture of the patient's symptoms, and family and medication history. Collecting routine medical information via a questionnaire allows staff to spend more time on patient and teaching activities, thus encouraging patients to become stimulated to assume a more active role in the encounter[9].

Practical example of a questionnaire

At the end of this chapter is a general health history questionnaire used by the house staff at Oakwood Hospital in Dearborn, Michigan (Figure 5-1) in conjunction with a dictation macro (Table 5-1). The questionnaire is given to the patient or family by the nursing staff either in the emergency room or on the general medical floor. We encourage the nursing staff to hand out the questionnaire by giving a pen or candy bar if the form is successfully completed. If the form is not completed the house staff or medical student will complete the form with the patient or family. Health history questionnaires may also be filled out on the telephone if the patient is unable, or members of his or her family are not in the hospital. Health history questionnaires are used in a similar fashion in the out-patient arena, except that we mail a copy of the form before the office visit.

The dictation macro

Also included in this chapter is a template for history dictation which is in our hospitals word processing system. We call this our 'history and physical' macro. This standardized format appears on the computer whenever the house officer announces that they want to use the history/dictation macro. Each house officer has a copy of the macro in their pocket so that they can follow a standardized format when they dictate. If they leave out information about a statement such as 'cardiopulmonary' in the review of systems, 'cardiopulmonary' will show up on the dictation with a blank space after it.

Table 5-1. Oakwood Hospital (Dearborn, Michigan) history and physical examination dictation macro

History

Chief complaint:

Present illness: This is a .... year old, admitted to Oakwood Hospital on ....

Current medications:

Past history:
    Past medical history —
    Past surgical/trauma history —
    Child illness —
    Drug allergy/toxicity/intolerance —

Family history:

Systematic review:
    General/endocrine/integument —
    Heent —
    Cardiorespiratory —
    Gastrointestinal —
    Musculoskeletal —
    Urological/reproductive —
    Neuropsychiatric —

Social and occupational history:
    Living situation —
    Sexual history —
    Tobacco consumption —
    Alcohol/drug use —
    Occupation history —

Physical examination

Vital signs:
General/integument:
Heent:
Neck:
Breasts:
Chest:
Cardiovascular:

(continued)

Table 5-1 (continued)

Abdomen:
Genitourinary:
Rectal:
Pelvic:
Extremities/back:
Neurological:

Laboratory

Impression

Plan

Dictated by:

Using a dictation macro reminds the house officer to be thorough. You will note that the health history questionnaire follows the same sequence as the dictation macro, thereby allowing an oral 'chief complaint and history of present illness', to be taken, and the health history questionnaire to be used in organizing routine family, past medical history, drugs, allergies and social history to improve the dictated records. The average time for dictation of a history and physical by one of the authors (Lyle Victor) is about 4.5–5 minutes.

CONCLUSION

The health history questionnaire and dictation macro are adjuncts to help collect and organize routine data thereby allowing the dictation of an excellent history and physical efficiently. The health history questionnaire is *not* a substitute for a thoughtful history of present illness and, in fact, in one study was inferior to the physician's ability to find subtle clues in the patient's history which would suggest serious disease[10].

The questionnaire saves time and collects much more data than the average history documented by house officers and attending physicians[11]. Having a completed form allows more time to be spent on the patient's current physical and emotional concerns. The health history questionnaire, while standardizing the medical information obtained, also helps develop communication, rapport, and patient education and compliance, without sacrificing the collection of complete historical data[12]. Used wisely the health history questionnaire and dictation macro will be able to save time and improve documentation quality.

REFERENCES

1. Institute of Medicine (1991). *The Computer-Based Patient Record: An Essential Technology for Health Care.* (Washington DC: National Academy Press)
2. Forkner, C. E. (1960). Record of medical history. *Arch. Intern. Med.,* **106,** 22–86
3. Dick, R. S. (1991). The Institute of Medicine's patient record study and its implications for record administrators. *Top Health Rec. Management,* **11,** 67–72
4. De Domball, F. T. (1978). Medical diagnoses from a clinician's point of view. *Meth. Inform. Med.,* **17,** 28–35
5. Joyce, C. R. B., Caple, G., Mason, M., Reynolds, E. and Mathews, J. A. (1969). Quantitative study of doctor–patient communication. *Q. J. Med. (new series),* **38,** 183–94
6. Mellner, C., Gardmark, S. and Parkholm, S. (1970). Medical questionnaires in clinical practice. In *Information Processing of Medical Records.* (Amsterdam: North Holland)
7. Victor, L. D. (ed.) (1992). *Clinical Pulmonary Medicine.* (Boston: Little, Brown and Co.)
8. Brondman, K., Erdmann, A. J., Lorge, I., Wolff, H. G. and Broadbent, T. H. (1949). The Cornell Medical Index — an adjunct to medical interview. *J. Am. Med. Assoc.,* **140,** 530–4
9. Inui, T. S. *et al.* (1979). Effects of a self-administered health history on new-patient visits in a general medical clinic. *Med. Care,* **17,** 1221–8
10. Hickam, D. H., Sox, H. C. and Sox, C. (1985). Systematic biases in recording the history in patients with chest pain. *J. Chronic Dis.,* 91–100
11. Victor, L. D. and Smolinski, M. (1991). Health History Questionnaires: Are they Useful? Poster presentation at the *36th Annual Scientific Meeting of the American College of Chest Physicians,* San Francisco
12. Pecoraro, R. E., Inui, T. S., Chen, M. S., Plorde, D. K. and Heller, J. L. (1979). Validity and reliability of a self-administered health history questionnaire. *Public Health Rep.,* **94,** 231–8

Figure 5-1. A general health history questionnaire used by house staff at Oakwood Hospital in Dearborn, Michigan

IMPORTANT!!
INFORMATION FOR YOUR HEALTH CARE PROVIDER

Dear Patient:

The following health history questionnaire will give important information to your health care providers. Please fill the form out as completely as possible.

If you have difficulty, please have a nurse or a family member assist you. A completed form will save your doctors from having to ask you many minutes worth of tedious questions and allow them to focus more on what you consider your main health problems.

Thank you

HEALTH HISTORY AND REVIEW OF SYSTEMS
Please answer all questions!

PATIENT NAME _____ AGE: _____ DATE: _____
IF SOMEONE OTHER THAN THE PATIENT HELPED FILL OUT THIS FORM:
WHAT IS YOUR NAME _____
RELATIONSHIP TO THE PATIENT _____
Chief complaint/history of present illness
What medical problem brought you to our hospital/clinic:

_____
_____
_____
_____
_____

Have you ever been evaluated at our hospital/clinic?   Yes _____ No _____ ? _____
When were you last seen at our hospital/clinic? _____

(continued)

LIST BELOW ANY MEDICINE YOU ARE NOW TAKING: CURRENT MEDICATIONS
(Please include all vitamins, aspirin, pain remedies, laxatives, tranquilizers and inhalers)

Name of medicine	Dose (mg, tsp, tbsp)	How often taken?	Date started

Do you use home oxygen? Yes ____ No ____ If so, how many liters per minute ____
If you need more space to list your medicines, use the back of this sheet.

PLEASE LIST ANY ALLERGIES OR REACTIONS TO MEDICINES

Name of medicine	Reaction (rash, wheezing, etc.)	Date

If you need more space to list your allergies or reactions to medicine,
please use the back of this sheet.

(continued)

LIST ANY OF YOUR PREVIOUS HOSPITALIZATIONS OR SURGERIES EXCEPT FOR NORMAL PREGNANCIES

Date(s)	Reason for hospitalization	Name/location	Name of doctor

LIST HERE ANY DOCTORS YOU HAVE SEEN IN THE PAST FIVE YEARS

Date	Reason	City	Name of doctor

(continued)

PAST MEDICAL AND FAMILY HISTORY

(Please place an X in box beside any of your illnesses or your families illnesses)

	Your illness	Mother	Father	Your grandparents (list by name)				Your children (list by name)					Your brothers/ sisters (list by name)				Your aunt/ uncle(s) (list by name)		
				1.	2.	3.	4.	1.	2.	3.	4.	5.	1.	2.	3.	4.	1.	2.	3.
Present age																			
Age at death (if deceased)																			
Cancer																			
Diabetes																			
High blood pressure																			
Heart attack																			
Angina																			
Rheumatic fever																			
Ulcers																			
Arthritis																			
Gout																			
Liver disease/ cirrhosis or yellow jaundice/ hepatitis																			
Allergies																			
Emphysema																			
Asthma																			
Tuberculosis																			
Convulsions (epilepsy/fits)																			
Nerve disease (polio/MS)																			
Alzheimer's																			
Stroke																			
Nervous breakdown																			
Suicide attempt																			
Drug abuse																			
Bleeding disorder																			
AIDS/exposed to AIDS																			
Gonorrhea																			
Syphilis																			

(continued)

PLACE AN X IN BOX BESIDE ANY OF YOUR MEDICAL PROBLEMS

Problem	Yes	No	Dates
Pneumonia:			
— How many times have you had pneumonia?_____			
— Date of last episode			
Bronchitis:			
— How many times have you had bronchitis?_____			
— Date of last episode			
Thrombophlebitis in legs (blood clots in the veins)			
Pulmonary embolus (blood clots in lung)			
Hiatal hernia			
Reflux esophagitis (heartburn)			
Black lung disease			
Childhood illnesses:			
— Measles			
— Chicken pox			
— Mumps			
— Whooping cough			
Thyroid problems:			
— Low thyroid			
— Hyperactive thyroid (overactive)			
Anemia (low blood)			
Heart murmur			
Blood transfusions			
Diverticulitis			
Colitis			
Migraine			
Glaucoma			
Cataracts			
Eczema			
Kidney stones			
Kidney infections			
Kidney failure/dialysis			

(continued)

REVIEW OF BODY SYSTEMS

	Yes	No	Unsure?

General; endocrine; skin

— Do you have a decreased appetite?...................................... Yes ____ No ____ ? ____
— Have you lost weight recently? .... Yes ____ No ____ ? ____
— Have you had a fever lately? .... Yes ____ No ____ ? ____
— Have you had chills lately? (The shakes or shivers) .... Yes ____ No ____ ? ____
— Do you sweat at night soaking your clothes or sheets? .... Yes ____ No ____ ? ____
— Do you have dry skin?.. Yes ____ No ____ ? ____
— Have you had a rash recently? .... Yes ____ No ____ ? ____
— Do you have any unusual lumps in your breasts?............. Yes ____ No ____ ? ____
— Have you had discharge from your nipples? .... Yes ____ No ____ ? ____
— Do you feel *hot* or *cold* when others are comfortable? ..... Yes ____ No ____ ? ____
— Have you had recent increase in thirst or appetite? .... Yes ____ No ____ ? ____
— Have you had any unusual hair growth or loss? .... Yes ____ No ____ ? ____

Heent

— Have you had blurred or double vision?............................ Yes ____ No ____ ? ____
— Do you have any blind spots in your vision? .... Yes ____ No ____ ? ____
— Do you have trouble hearing? .... Yes ____ No ____ ? ____
— Do you have ringing or roaring in your ears?.................... Yes ____ No ____ ? ____
— Do you have frequent nosebleeds? .... Yes ____ No ____ ? ____
— Do you have soreness in your mouth or tongue? .... Yes ____ No ____ ? ____
— Do you have difficulty swallowing? .... Yes ____ No ____ ? ____
— Do you have hoarseness or change in your voice? .... Yes ____ No ____ ? ____
— Do you cough or choke when you drink or eat?................ Yes ____ No ____ ? ____
— Have you had a sore throat recently?................................ Yes ____ No ____ ? ____
— Have you had a runny nose recently?................................ Yes ____ No ____ ? ____
— Have you had an earache recently? .... Yes ____ No ____ ? ____

Cardiorespiratory

— Do you cough? .... Yes ____ No ____ ? ____
— Do you cough up phlegm? .... Yes ____ No ____ ? ____
— Do you have shortness of breath?...................................... Yes ____ No ____ ? ____
— Do you wake up at night wheezing or short of breath?.... Yes ____ No ____ ? ____
— How many pillows do you sleep on?
    Check: ( )one ( )two ( )three ( )four
— Do you wheeze or make musical sounds
    when you breathe? .... Yes ____ No ____ ? ____
— Have you coughed up blood? .... Yes ____ No ____ ? ____
— When was your last skin test for tuberculosis (TB):
    Date _____ *Reaction:* Check: ( )positive? ( )negative?

(continued)

— Do you have palpitations or unusual beats of your heart? Yes ____ No ____ ? ____
— Do you ever get chest pain or discomfort?......................... Yes ____ No ____ ? ____
    If yes, is the discomfort: Check all that apply:
      ( )aching?; ( )sharp?; ( )dull?; ( )burning?;
      ( )pressing or constricting?

If you have chest pain please answer ALL of the following questions:
    — Do you get chest discomfort when you exercise? .... Yes ____ No ____ ? ____
    — Does the chest discomfort increase with breathing? .. Yes ____ No ____ ? ____
    — Does the chest pain increase with cough? .... Yes ____ No ____ ? ____
    — Does the chest discomfort go into your:
      Check: ( )jaw?; ( )arm?; ( )back? .... Yes ____ No ____ ? ____
    — Was your chest pain ever evaluated by a doctor?....... Yes ____ No ____ ? ____
      If so, when and what was the diagnosis_____
— Do you have swollen ankles?... Yes ____ No ____ ? ____
— Do you have cramps at rest or while walking?................. Yes ____ No ____ ? ____

Gastrointestinal

— Do you often feel sick to your stomach or nauseated?...... Yes ____ No ____ ? ____
— Have you ever vomited blood or material that looked
    like coffee grounds?... Yes ____ No ____ ? ____
— Do you get pain or discomfort in your stomach? .... Yes ____ No ____ ? ____
— Have you had a recent change in your bowel habits?...... Yes ____ No ____ ? ____
— Are you often constipated? .... Yes ____ No ____ ? ____
— Do you have pain in your rectum? .... Yes ____ No ____ ? ____
— Do you have loose or watery bowel movements? .... Yes ____ No ____ ? ____
— Have you noticed black or tar colored bowel movements? Yes ____ No ____ ? ____
— Have you had pencil thin bowel movements?.................... Yes ____ No ____ ? ____

Musculoskeletal

— Do you have swelling or redness of your joints?................. Yes ____ No ____ ? ____
— Have you had pain in any of your joints or spine? .... Yes ____ No ____ ? ____
— Have you had limitation of your joints or spine?................ Yes ____ No ____ ? ____

Urological/reproductive

— Have you had cloudy or foul smelling urine ('pee')? .... Yes ____ No ____ ? ____
— Has your urine been red or tea colored? .... Yes ____ No ____ ? ____
— Do you get up more than once a night to urinate?............. Yes ____ No ____ ? ____
— Do you have pain or burning when you urinate? .... Yes ____ No ____ ? ____
— Do you have trouble starting or stopping urination?.......... Yes ____ No ____ ? ____
— Do you have the feeling that you must urinate,
    but pass only small amounts of urine? .... Yes ____ No ____ ? ____

(continued)

For women only

— Do you have abnormal vaginal bleeding? .... Yes ____ No ____ ? ____

— What was the date of your first menstrual period?_____

— What was the date of your last menstrual period?_____

     Is your menstrual flow heavier than previously?............. Yes ____ No ____ ? ____

— Did you have high blood pressure with any of

     your pregnancies?... Yes ____ No ____ ? ____

— Did you have high blood sugar or diabetes during

     any of your pregnancies? .... Yes ____ No ____ ? ____

For men only

— Do you have any pain or lumps in your testicles?............... Yes ____ No ____ ? ____

— Is your urinary stream weaker that it used to be?.............. Yes ____ No ____ ? ____

— Do you have discharge from your penis? .... Yes ____ No ____ ? ____

— Have you ever had homosexual contact?............................ Yes ____ No ____ ? ____

Neuropsychiatric

— Are you troubled by frequent headaches?......................... Yes ____ No ____ ? ____

— Are there times when everything seems to spin? .... Yes ____ No ____ ? ____

— Are there times when you feel faint or lightheaded? .... Yes ____ No ____ ? ____

— Have you had any unusual shaking of your hands?......... Yes ____ No ____ ? ____

— Have you had any difficulty walking? .... Yes ____ No ____ ? ____

— Have you had a recent change in your speech?............... Yes ____ No ____ ? ____

— Have you had fainting or blackout spells lately? .... Yes ____ No ____ ? ____

— Are you depressed? .... Yes ____ No ____ ? ____

— Do you often feel like crying?.. Yes ____ No ____ ? ____

— Has life ever seemed so difficult that you seriously

     wanted to end it all? .... Yes ____ No ____ ? ____

— Are you excessively sleepy? .... Yes ____ No ____ ? ____

— Do you have trouble sleeping? .... Yes ____ No ____ ? ____

— Have you ever fallen asleep while driving? .... Yes ____ No ____ ? ____

— Do people complain about your snoring? .... Yes ____ No ____ ? ____

— Have you *ever* seen a psychiatrist or counselor? .... Yes ____ No ____ ? ____

— Have you *ever* been told by your doctor or psychiatrist

     that you have any of the following illnesses:

        Check where appropriate

        ( ) depression?;   ( ) manic/depression?;

        ( ) schizophrenia?; ( ) nervous exhaustion?;

        ( ) panic disorder?; ( ) chronic anxiety disorder?

(continued)

HAVE YOU HAD ANY OF THE FOLLOWING LAB TESTS
IN THE PAST FIVE (5) YEARS?

Test	What hospital or clinic	Ordering doctor	Date of exam
Gastrointestinal series			
CAT scan of chest			
CAT scan of abdomen			
MRI exam of head			
Blood count			
Blood chemistry			
Barium enema			
Colonoscopy			
Holter monitor (device to check your heart beat for 24 hours)			
Bronchoscopy (lighted tube to look at chest and lungs)			
Chest tube (to obtain fluid or air from your chest)			
Pulmonary function tests			
Gastroscopy (lighted tube to look at the stomach)			
Mammogram			
2D echocardiogram (probe placed on the heart)			
Nuclear scan of heart (MUGA)			

SOCIAL AND OCCUPATIONAL/WORK HISTORY
(Please answer all questions)

Marital status: unmarried   married   divorced   widowed   (please circle one)

How many times have you been married?_____

Religious preference (optional) _____

Residences (state or country): Location(s) as a child-_____

Location(s) as an adult-_____

Present living situation: check: (   ) with family; (   ) relatives; (   ) friends;

(   ) nursing home; (   ) alone

	Yes	No	Unsure

— Do you drive a car? .... Yes ____No ____ ? ____

If not, please explain_____

(continued)

— Have you *ever* smoked cigarettes?.................................. Yes ____ No ____ ? ____
    If yes:
    How old were you when you had your first cigarette?___
    When did you have your last cigarette?_____
    How old were you when you had your last cigarette?___
    How many packs of cigarettes per day did you smoke
        when you smoked the most? _____
— Have you *ever* smoked a pipe?.. Yes ____ No ____ ? ____
— Have you *ever* smoked cigars?... Yes ____ No ____ ? ____
— How many drinks containing alcohol do you drink in a
    24 hour period?   Weekday   Weekend
     Cans of beer   _____   _____
     Glasses of wine   _____   _____
     Shots of liquor   _____   _____
— When was your last alcoholic drink? (date) _____
— Do you ever drink in the morning to calm your nerves or
    to 'get yourself going'? .... Yes ____ No ____ ? ____
— Have you ever attended an 'AA' (Alcoholics Anonymous)
    or Alanon meeting? .... Yes ____ No ____ ? ____
— Have you ever had a drunk driving charge?.................... Yes ____ No ____ ? ____
— Do you think you drink too much or feel guilty about
    drinking? .... Yes ____ No ____ ? ____
— How many cups of coffee do you drink per day?
    ( ) Regular ( ) Decaf.
— How many cups of tea do you drink per day?
    ( ) Regular ( ) Decaf.
— Have you ever used the following drugs?
    Check: ( ) sleeping pills?; ( ) heroin?; ( ) cocaine?;
             ( ) diet pills?; ( ) marijuana?
— What is, or was your main line of work _____
— What is, or was your spouses main line of work _____
— If you are not presently working: Check one or more:
    ( ) Are you retired?; ( ) are you laid off?;
    ( ) have you been recently fired?;
    ( ) do you receive workman's compensation?;
    ( ) are you on disability?
    Date any of the above stated_____

(continued)

— If you are on workman's compensation or disability,
   please list the reason(s): _____
   _____

— Have you ever had problems with the police or law?......... Yes ____ No ____ ? ____
   If yes, what was the reason: _____
   _____

— Do you work around any hazardous material? .... Yes ____ No ____ ? ____
   If so, what is it?_____

— Do you have any pets? .... Yes ____ No ____ ? ____
   If yes, please desribe_____

— If you have traveled outside the United States in the
   past two years, please list places:_____
   _____

IF YOU HAVE HAD ANY OF THESE JOBS/CLASSIFICATIONS, PLEASE CHECK ( ):

( ) Asbestos worker   ( ) Foundryman   ( ) Sandblaster
( ) Auto mechanic   ( ) Glass maker   ( ) Ship builder
( ) Brake worker   ( ) Grinder   ( ) Stone worker
( ) Brick maker/layer   ( ) Insulation worker   ( ) Sugar cane worker
( ) Carpenter   ( ) Mill worker   ( ) Wall board worker
( ) Coal miner   ( ) Miner   ( ) Welder
( ) Construction worker ( ) Polisher
( ) Flame cutter   ( ) Roofer

6

Sleep and shift work

L. D. Victor

INTRODUCTION

Interns and residents are often sleep-deprived shift workers. Irregular sleep and work schedules often impact adversely on a house officer's mood and ability to perform tasks that require constant vigilance. This chapter offers strategies that will help residents in optimizing their work performance and sense of well-being in a chronically sleep-deprived state.

NORMAL SLEEP

No one knows for certain why humans must sleep. Many authorities recognize it as a biological need that, if unmet, causes the pursuit of sleep in a similar manner as we might for food and water. Most adults need between 7 and 9 hours of sleep a night. Physiologically short sleepers may need only 4 or 5 hours and feel and function perfectly normally, whereas physiologically long sleepers may need up to 9 or more hours a night to avoid symptoms of sleep deprivation. I suspect that surgeons and emergency room physicians are often people that require relatively less sleep as opposed to someone like myself (a sleep specialist and program director), or perhaps a psychiatrist, who may discover early in medical school that their sleep requirements are higher. Other individuals avoid work situations that disrupt sleep, finding that the dysphoria the next day is debilitating. Sleep requirements are biologically determined and are not a function of someone's ambition and drive for success.

Stages of sleep

In medical school you learned that there are sleep stages 1–4 and rapid eye movement (REM or dream) sleep. Stage 1 is the lightest state of sleep during which time you can be easily aroused, as is true with REM sleep. As the progression occurs through stage 2 and stages 3 and 4 (slow wave or delta) sleep, arousability becomes increasingly more difficult. Slow wave sleep is thought to be the most restorative sleep. A normal sleeper will initiate sleep through stage 1 and move through the various stages of sleep in an orderly fashion throughout the night in four or five cycles. Most slow wave sleep occurs during the first part of the night, whereas most REM sleep occurs in the early morning hours just prior to awakening. Penile tumescence occurs in normal males during REM sleep.

Implications of the different sleep stages

Sleep stages have important implications for house officers as your ability to awaken and think clearly is dependent on this. For example, if you are aroused just after you go to bed in the early part of the night, the chances are good that you will be in the deeper, slow wave sleep and will have difficulty awakening. Slow wave sleep is associated with the so-called sleep inertia[1,2], when cognition and memory may be impaired up to 15 minutes. Rapid eye movement sleep arousals are associated with less impairment than slow wave sleep awakenings[1,3]. Arousal from sleep also may affect event recall as short-term memory is lost if you are not awake for more than 5 minutes before falling back to sleep again. These facts have important implications for patient care as it is entirely possible to receive critical patient information and give orders and have no memory of these events in the morning[4].

CIRCADIAN RHYTHMS

In the sixteenth century De Marain discovered that the mimosa plant would open and close its leaves to receive sun in a periodic fashion throughout the day, even in a darkened closet. Since then many biological rhythms have been described such as menstruation, which occurs with a regular periodicity of about a month. Circadian rhythms are those biological rhythms with a periodicity of about a day (from the Greek *circa* meaning about and *dias* meaning day). The sleep/wake cycle is a circadian rhythm. Birth and death are also circadian rhythms, both having a tendency to occur in the early morning hours. Sudden cardiac death[5] and stroke[6] usually occur between 6.00 a.m. and 12.00 noon and thus may be considered circadian.

Human sleep/wake rhythms

The human biological clock may be studied in situations of temporal isolation. Humans kept in this situation, without clocks or daylight, exhibit an endogenous and self-sustaining rhythm of sleep and wakefulness[7]. Under these circumstances, the days and nights gradually get longer and longer. Circadian rhythm researchers have shown that the period of the human sleep/wake cycle is about 25 hours. The natural tendency for the human biological clock is to make the day longer or to stay up later and later. This fact explains why jet lag is less severe when traveling westward thorough multiple time zones, when it is necessary to stay up later. It is much more difficult for humans to go to bed earlier, as is required when traveling through multiple time zones in the easterly direction; this is often the situation when going to Europe from the United States.

Resetting the biological clock

Each day, on awakening, we reset the biological clock by opening our eyes to daylight, thereby keeping us 'entrained' to a 24-hour day. Zeitgebers (time givers) are the agents of change for biological rhythms. The major zeitgeber for humans is daylight streaming through open eyes. Other possible zeitgebers include social interaction and meals. The actual biological clock is thought to be a small cluster of cells in the superchiasmic nucleus[8,9]. Because of the natural inclination for the biological clock to reset itself later and later each day, it stands to reason that it is easier for us to force ourselves to stay up later, rather than go to bed earlier. For most people, 2 or 3 hours is not too difficult to phase delay the day (stay up later). Going to bed earlier, or phase advancing the day, is much more difficult; most people have problems attempting their nocturnal sleep period earlier than an hour before their usual bedtime, unless they are sleep deprived. Think about it; is it easier to stay up 2 hours later or go to bed an hour earlier?

Body temperature and sleeping

Body temperature is a biological rhythm tied to sleepiness and alertness. For example, most people choose to go to bed around the peak of body temperature and sleep through a time of the lowest body temperature, around 4.00 or 5.00 a.m. Awakening usually occurs just after the body temperature starts to rise. Body temperature begins to level off in the mid-afternoon and is associated with a time of increased sleepiness (post-lunch dip), then starts to increase again in the early evening, which coincides with a period of increased alertness (evening wake maintenance zone). Researchers often measure body temperature as a means of identifying changes in circadian rhythms and adaptation to time changes during studies on jet lag.

'Owls' and 'larks'

People who are 'larks' tend to be early risers, are very alert early in the day and require an early bedtime. 'Owls' on the other hand, have difficulty getting up in the morning, but their level of alertness increases as the day progresses and peaks in the evening hours; they tend to be most alert at midnight. The level of alertness in 'larks' and 'owls' may be related to body temperature curves. However, owls have an excellent capacity to sleep late, even into the morning 'wake up zone' from 9.00 to 11.00 a.m. predicted by rising body temperature and circadian physiology.

The natural aging process tends to make us larks[10] as we get older, with early sleep and awake times being common in the elderly.

It should be noted that owls do tend to function better during periods of irregular sleep/wake schedules than do larks.

Sleep latency

Researchers have studied the effect of a series of naps throughout the day and measured the time to sleep onset (sleep latency). Normal adults will take about 10 minutes to fall asleep. Sleep-deprived persons or those with circadian difficulties may have latencies to sleep of a couple of minutes or less. Almost everyone has increased sleepiness, or reduced time to sleep onset, in the mid-afternoon and increased alertness around 11.00 a.m. and between 6.00 and 8.00 p.m., the so-called morning and evening wake maintenance zones[11]. These alert and sleepy periods have important implications for task performance. Automobile accidents in Israel occurred more often at night and around the 3.00 p.m. dip[12]. Resident performance for monotonous tasks may be impaired at these times, even if there is no sleep deprivation.

JET LAG

Jet lag is just a consequence of trying to defy human circadian physiology. Humans have the capability to delay sleep onset for 2 or 3 hours or advance sleep onset by 30–60 minutes without too much difficulty. Problems arise when the international traveler starts to journey through several time zones.

Traveling east

Easterly travel is much more difficult because the traveler must force themselves to go to bed earlier. For example, most flights going to Europe leave at night, arriving the next morning, which is essentially 1.00 or 2.00 a.m. for the traveler. By the time you get through customs and to your room, it may be 4.00 or 5.00 a.m. to the traveler and about 1.00 p.m. local time. If the traveler attempts to sleep, they will wake up after only a few hours as their circadian system approaches the morning wake up zone with its rapid rise in body temperature. The bedtime in the new time zone presents the biggest problem for the easterly traveler's biological clock, because when it is 11.00 p.m. in Europe it is only 6.00 p.m. New York time. There is no way the biological clock can advance by that many hours and insomnia follows. From a practical standpoint, the first nights sleep after traveling to Europe may not be all that bad because of the significant sleep deprivation from the trip, as it is almost impossible to get uninterrupted sleep on an airplane. The following night may be associated with severe insomnia. When traveling to Europe it is best to go out into bright sunlight and reset the biological clock. Adding bright light towards the end of a sleep period will tend to cause a phase advance (ability to go to sleep earlier).

Traveling west

Westward travel is easier because it is more compatible with the natural tendency for the biological clock to delay sleep onset. Travelers in both directions tend to have 'terminal insomnia,' that is, an early wake up time and an inability to have a normal, uninterrupted sleep for 7 or 8 hours, because in either direction the sleeper is confronted with the biological clock's morning wake up zone or evening wake maintenance zone. However, a 7- or 9-hour time zone change in an easterly direction will require 8–12 days to accommodate, whereas only a 5–7 day acclimatization period may be necessary in the westward direction.

SLEEP DEPRIVATION

Most adults are slightly sleep deprived, but suffer few adverse consequences. It is possible to miss an entire night's sleep without a great reduction in performance the next day. The next night's sleep (recovery sleep) will be deeper, showing a generous amount of slow wave sleep; REM sleep recovers during the ensuing nights.

Chronic sleep deprivation

Problems begin when there is significant chronic sleep deprivation. Given the nocturnal work schedules of primary care residents, there is every reason to believe that they are in this chronically sleep-deprived category. Studies have shown that tasks of short duration requiring a high level of attention and motor capability (e.g. intubation) appear to be preserved[13], whereas those that are monotonous, but require constant vigilance, might be impaired[14,15]. In addition, the excessively sleepy person may suffer from micro-sleeps during the day, manifested by brief (less than 20 seconds) bursts of electroencephalograph (EEG) sleep activity. This may impair attention span and memory. Some researchers believe that the very act of resisting sleep in the sleep-deprived state uses sufficient energy to reduce performance[16].

Measurement of sleepiness

An objective measure of sleepiness is provided by the multiple sleep latency test (MSLT)[17]; this has shown that the normal individual, on average, will take more than 10 minutes to fall asleep whereas subjects that are pathologically sleepy will drift into sleep in less than 5 minutes[18].

Sleep-deprived persons are not good predictors of how sleepy they are. One researcher reported zero correlation between a self-administered questionnaire and sleep latency documented by the MSLT[19]. One reason for this may be that the sensation of sleepiness can be hard to interpret, with sleepy individuals complaining of tiredness, lack of energy, or memory and concentration problems instead. Another way to gage sleepiness is how easily you tend to nap during boring, monotonous situations such as reading medical textbooks, watching television, driving or sitting in the opera. These situations do not 'put you to sleep,' but allow sleep to occur more readily in the already sleepy person.

The sleep-deprived person who also is a shift worker, as house officers are, is confronted with even greater problems. Your situation may be equivalent to an insufficient sleeper who also is suffering from jet lag.

Sleep disruption

Sleep disruption can be just as deleterious as deprivation. One study showed that disruptions that caused arousal from sleep at 1-minute intervals but with a normal total sleep time were as bad as no sleep at all. However, they also demonstrated that reasonable performance the next day could be maintained if the subjects were allowed to obtain at least

10 minutes of sleep before interruptions[20]. Another study reported that interruptions occurring over a series of sleep nights were even more deleterious to performance the next day[21]. These data suggest that the house officer's often random sleep disruptions may result in impaired performance the next day because of a lack of sleep continuity.

SHIFT WORK

As a house officer, you are part of the 20% of the working population who must work on shifts other than 9.00 a.m. to 5.00 p.m. Your problem is compounded because you must work over long time periods, being expected to maintain excellent vigilance for 36 or more hours; a requirement that counters circadian physiology and good sleep hygiene. Factors that may be associated with difficulty performing shift work include: older age, moonlighting and heavy domestic responsibilities (especially true for women with children). Other important factors include being a 'lark,' having previous sleep problems, substance abuse, and major medical problems such as diabetes and heart disease[22].

Shift workers average less sleep than daytime workers. For example, permanent night workers will average about an hour less per night than their counterparts working during the day[23]. Workers starting their work day at unusually early hours, such as at 5.00 a.m., also may suffer from insufficient sleep[24]. Such an early work time would require the shift worker to go to bed around 8.00 p.m. in order to get a standard 8 hours sleep, a very difficult task in modern society. Because of irregular sleeping and waking schedules, shift workers suffer both from insomnia when they want to sleep and excessive sleepiness and fatigue when they want to work. Sleepiness may impair job performance and contribute to the cause of severe accidents such as airplane crashes[25] and nuclear accidents[26]. Sleep on the job has been documented in the form of intrusions of sleep EEG rhythms in the θ range in some night workers[27].

SLEEP STRATEGIES FOR THE SLEEP-DEPRIVED SHIFT WORKER (THAT'S YOU!)

Obviously, you should attempt to get sufficient sleep on your nights off. How much you need is biologically determined, but is seldom less than 7–8 hours a night unless you are a physiologically short sleeper. Exercising good sleep hygiene when you do sleep is important. Consider the following tips:

(1) Go to bed and wake up at the same time each day, even on the weekends. The wake up time resets the biological clock and is even more important than the time of sleep onset. Insomniacs often have random wake up times.

(2) Use the bed only for sleep and sex. The bedroom is a poor place for marital arguments.

(3) Avoid 'tossing and turning' in bed. If you cannot fall asleep in 20–30 minutes, leave the bedroom until drowsy. Reading medical journals has a more soporific effect than benzodiazepines!

(4) Exercise often, but not in the evening if this interferes with sleep. Trained athletes have more of the restorative slow wave sleep after exercising. Untrained athletes may have difficulty sleeping after a bout of vigorous exercise.

(5) Excess alcohol causes problems. Alcoholic beverages are particularly dangerous in the sleep-deprived individual as they shorten sleep latency considerably, and although it may be easier to fall asleep, there are more arousals during the night. In addition, there may be difficulty falling back to sleep when awakening from REM sleep.

(6) Caffeine can hurt or help the sleepy resident. Using coffee to stay awake during the night may well interfere with attempts to sleep during the next day. Overuse of caffeine is a particular problem for the 'night float' team member who must sleep during the daytime hours after working all night.

Using knowledge of circadian physiology can be of great use to residents working night hours. For example, the longer the time of sleep deprivation, up to 32 hours in one study, the shorter the subsequent sleep period. The shortest sleep times occurred when the subject attempted sleep in the late morning or noon[28], corresponding to the circadian wake up period. In time isolation experiments subjects rarely choose to initiate sleep during these times[29]. The use of sleeping pills[30] or alcohol to initiate sleep is ill-advised. The resident who is up all night would be better off staying awake until early afternoon before attempting sleep in order to benefit from the post-lunch dip in alertness and circadian increase in sleepiness in the mid-afternoon as body temperature begins to flatten out. If you are up all night, consider trying to finish your work before the afternoon in order to avoid severe sleepiness. Another way to think about this is the following: the day shift worker has an 'evening' period to eat and relax before attempting to sleep. The night shift worker should consider having an 'evening' in which to wind down, but this will be during the morning. Come home, have breakfast, relax, and sleep at mid-day. A corollary to this is a useful practice I learned from the evening shift (4.00–11.00 p.m.) workers, who frequently give themselves time to wind down and reduce adrenaline levels. Most evening shift workers who leave work at 11.00 p.m. will eat and relax before attempting sleep at 2.00 or 3.00 a.m.

Many training programs have a night float system where a group of residents will work only at night and sleep during the day. Initially the day sleep will be shorter with increased disruptions in the latter third of the sleep period[31]. Poor quality sleep will continue for up to 2 or more weeks. Another problem of many night shift workers is that they revert to a daytime activity cycle on their days off; this may also prolong acclimatization to a nocturnal schedule.

Napping can be extremely useful for the resident having to work long hours. Napping is very common among nocturnal workers[32], and may be involuntary while in the upright position[33]. Some subjects find naps counterproductive, so each shift worker has to determine whether it is beneficial for him or her. Certainly napping has improved performance during prolonged periods of sleep deprivation and arduous work[34]. Some shift workers benefit from a short nap in the afternoon prior to working all night. Naps during this time have a greater propensity for having slow wave sleep and hence will be more restorative, even if short. Be aware, however, that the slow wave sleep may increase your propensity for sleep inertia when napping at that time. Napping during the nocturnal work period may also be of use, especially during the most sleepy times around 4.00–5.00 a.m. Napping at this time may increase alertness the next day.

CONCLUSIONS
Internship and residency presents a difficult combination of challenging work in a sleep deprived state. Applying good sleep hygiene and circadian principles can reduce sleepiness and improve performance.

REFERENCES

1. Stones, M. J. (1977). Memory performance after arousal from different sleep stages. *Br. J. Psychol.*, **68**, 177–81
2. Langdon, D. E. and Hartmean, B. (1961). *Performance upon Sudden Awakening*, SAM report 62–17. (Brooks Air Force Base, Texas: US Air Force School of Aerospace Medicine)
3. Bonnet, M. H. (1993). Memory for events occurring during arousal from sleep. *Psychophysiology*, **20**, 81–7
4. Guilleminault, C. and Dement, W. C. (1977). Amnesia and disorders of excessive daytime sleepiness. In Drucker-Colin, R. R. and McGaugh, J. L. (eds.). *Neurobiology of Sleep and Memory*, pp. 439–56. (New York: Academic Press)
5. Muller, J. E., Ludmen, P. L., Willich, S. N., Fofler, G. H., Aylmer, G., Klangos, I. and Stone, P. H. (1987). Circadian variation in the frequency of sudden cardiac death. *Circulation*, **75**, 131
6. Tsementzis, S. A., Gill, F. S., Hitchcock, E. R., Gill, S. K. and Beevers, D. G. (1985). Diurnal variation of and activity during the onset of stroke. *Neurosurgery*, **17**, 901–4
7. Wever, R. (1975). The circadian multi-oscillatory system of man. *Int. J. Chronobiol.*, **3**, 19–55
8. Daan, S., Beersma, D. G. M. and Borbely, A. A. (1984). Timing of human sleep: recovery process gated by a circadian pacemaker. *Am. J. Physiol.*, **246**, R161–78
9. Moore, R. Y. (1990). The circadian timing system and the organization of sleep-wake behavior. In Thorpy, M. J. (ed.) *Handbook of Sleep Disorders*, pp. 103–15. (New York: Marcel Dekker Inc.)
10. Tune, G. S. (1969). The influence of age and temperament on the adult human sleep-wakefulness pattern. *Br. J. Psychiatry*, **60**, 431–41
11. Strogatz, S. H., Kronauer, R. E. and Czeisler, C. A. (1987). Circadian pacemaker interferes with sleep onset at specific time each day. *Am. J. Physiol.*, **253**, R1–7
12. Lavie, P., Wollman, M. and Pollack, I. (1986). Frequency of sleep related traffic accidents and hour of the day. *Sleep Res.*, **15**, 275
13. Storer, J. S., Floyd, H. H., Gill, W. L., Guisti, C. W. and Ginsberg, H. (1989). Effects of sleep deprivation on cognitive ability and skills of pediatrics residents. *Acad. Med.*, **64**, 29–32
14. Friedman, R. C., Bigger, T. J. and Kornfeld, D. S. (1971). The intern and sleep loss. *N. Engl. J. Med.*, **285**, 202–3
15. Denisco, R. A., Drummond, D. and Gravenstein, J. S. (1987). The effect of fatigue on the performance of a simulated anesthetic monitoring task. *J. Clin. Monit.*, **3**, 22–4

16. Lavie, P., Gopher, D. and Wollman, M. (1987). Thirty-six hour correspondence between performance and sleepiness cycles. *Psychophysiology*, **3,** 22–4

17. Carskadon, M. A. and Bement, W. C. (1977). Sleep tendency: an objective measure of sleep loss. *Sleep Res.*, **6,** 200

18. Roth, T., Roehrs, T., Carskadon, M. and Dement, W. (1989). Daytime sleepiness and alertness. In Kryger, M., Roth, T. and Dement, W. (eds.) *Principles and Practice of Sleep Medicine*, pp. 14–23. (Philadelphia: W. B. Saunders)

19. Graeber, C. (1990). Circadian rhythm and jet lag. Oral presentation on the *Sleep Medicine and Technology Training and Education Center Course*, Stanford University

20. Bonnet, M. H. (1986). Performance and sleepiness as a function of frequency and placement of sleep disruption. *Psychophysiology*, **23,** 263–71

21. Bonnet, M. H. (1985). Effect of sleep disruption on sleep, performance and mood. *Sleep*, **8,** 1–9

22. Tepas, D. I. and Monk, T. H. (1987). Work schedules. In Salvendy, G. (ed.) *Handbook of Human Factors*, pp. 819–43. (New York: John Wiley and Sons)

23. Tepas, D. I., Walsh, J. K. and Armstrong, D. R. (1981). Comprehensive study of the sleep of shift workers. In Johnson, J. C., Tepas, D. I., Colquhoun, W. O. and Colligan, M. J. (eds.) *The Twenty-four Hour Workday. Proceedings of a Symposium on Variations in the Work-Sleep Schedules*, publication no. 81–127, pp. 419–34. (Washington, DC: Department of Health and Human Services (National Institute for Occupational Health and Safety))

24. Reinberg, A., Chaumont, A. and Laporte, A. (1975). Circadian temporal structure of 20 shift workers (8 hour shift-weekly rotation): an autometric field study. In Colquhour, W. P., Folkard, S., Knauth, P. and Rutenfranz, J. (eds.) *Experimental Studies of Shiftwork*, Forschungsberichte des Landes NRW Nr. 2513, pp. 142–65. (Opladen: Westdeutscher Verlag)

25. Price, W. J. and Holley, D. C. (1981). The last minutes of flight 2860: an analysis of crew shift work scheduling. In Reinberg, A. N., Vieus, N. and Andlauer, P. (eds.) *Night and Shift Work — Biological and Social Aspects*, pp. 287–94. (Oxford: Pergamon Press)

26. Hauri, P. and Linde, S. (1990). No more sleepless nights. In *Night Work, Jet Lag and Seasonal Affective Disorder*, pp. 148–58. (New York: John Wiley)

27. Torsvall, L. and Åkerstedt, F. (1980). Sleepiness on the job; continuously measured EEG changes in train drivers. *Electroencephalogr. Clin. Neurophysiol.*, **66,** 502–11

28. Åkerstedt, F. and Gillberg, M. (1981). The circadian variation of experimentally displaced sleep. *Sleep*, **4**, 159–69

29. Strogatz, S. H., Kronauer, R. E. and Czeisler, C. A. (1985). Circadian pacemaker interferes with sleep onset at specific time each day. *Sleep Res.*, **14**, 291

30. Walsh, J. K., Muehlbach, M. J. and Schweitzer, P. K. (1984). Acute administration of Trazolam for the daytime sleep of rotating shift workers. *Sleep*, **7**, 223–9

31. Weitzman, E. D., Kripke, D. F., Goldmacher, D., McGregor, P. and Nogeire, C. (1970). Acute reversal of the sleep–waking cycle in man; effect on sleep stage patterns. *Arch. Neurol.*, **22**, 483–9

32. Andersen, J. E. (1970). *Three-shift Work — A Socio-Medico–Investigation*, Vol. 1, pp. 134–59. (Copenhagen: Teknisk Forlag)

33. Kogi, K. (1981). Comparison of resting conditions between various shift rotation systems for industrial workers. In Reinberg, A. N., Vieux, N. and Andlauer, P. (eds.) *Night and Shift Work — Biological and Social Aspects*, pp. 155–60. (Oxford: Pergamon Press)

34. Opstad, P. K., Ekanger, R., Nummestad, M. and Raabe, N. (1978). Performance, mood and clinical symptoms in men exposed to prolonged, severe physical work and sleep deprivation. *Aviat. Space Environ. Med.*, **49**, 1065–73

7

Emotional survival in residency

S. D. Fabick

INTRODUCTION
Your residency is a time of great professional and personal challenge. As is true of any challenging time, significant emotional growth can result. This chapter addresses some of the psychological factors which are central to successful adjustment in residency. Among them are the ability to tolerate frustration and other aspects of ego-strength, setting broad and realistic goals, and, finally, stress reduction methods.

TOLERATING FRUSTRATION
In an effort to motivate you, someone may have said 'shoot for the moon and even if you fail, you will at least end up among the stars.' This advice may not only reflect an incomplete knowledge of astronomy, but of psychology as well.

Self-evaluation

Resources and ability. You should size up your chances for success before trying to achieve something. You estimate the requirements of what you aspire to and compare it with your own resources. You then make a decision about whether to try to achieve it. Furthermore, if you do decide to pursue it, you determine how you will go about the venture, how much time and energy to invest in it, and how much to disclose your intentions to others. For example, you gauge the intellectual demands of medical training with your own intellectual ability, consider your own attractiveness as you size up who to ask for a date, and try to match your qualifications with jobs you seek.

Capacity for disappointment. In addition, even if you are not aware of it, you take into account your estimate of your own capacity to experience disappointment. This is the fundamentally important part of striving ignored by the 'shoot for the moon' advice.

Ego-strength. Ego-strength is the psychological term for the capacity to experience disappointment and failure without a significant drop in mood and self-esteem (a subjective sense of worth). So the higher your ego-strength, the higher your sense of well-being, other things being equal. Ego-strength is like money in the bank. You not only feel more secure, but you also can invest (risk) more because of your reserves. As is true with money, it takes a certain amount of ego-strength in order to have a better chance to get more of the venture.

Ego-investment. Another pertinent factor in considering how much you can invest of yourself into striving for a goal, is how ego-invested you are in it (i.e. the extent your sense of self is tied to achieving the goal). For example, if a significant portion of your identity is related to your professional success, it will not only increase your desire to achieve that goal, but concomitantly raise the risk of depleting your sense of well-being if you end up seeing yourself as failing.

Beginner's luck represents a resolution of this dilemma. You expect very little of yourself the first time you try something, so you can often optimize your efforts (e.g. try very hard, but remain patient and relaxed). You can revive your beginner's luck each spring in your first golf outing. However, your raised expectations of yourself on subsequent outings quickly undermine the efficacy of this resolution of the problem.

Degree of determination. So how much you strive for a goal is based upon several variables such as your ability in a certain area, the level of ego-investment you have in attaining a goal, and circumstantial factors such as temporarily lowered expectations involved in something like beginner's luck, etc., and one constant which is your level of ego-strength.

What determines ego-strength?

Ego-strength is the product of many things, including your genetic endowment temperamentally, intellectually and physically. Perhaps more importantly, however, it is the imprint of your experiences, particularly related to disappointment, failure and uncertainty. Your earliest experiences and those with people you depended upon most (by definition this often overlaps greatly) have the greatest impact in the development of ego-strength. For example, the capacity to tolerate frustration develops best if there is generally reliable acceptance of the child's feelings and, without overindulgence, satisfaction of the child's needs by caretakers, typically parents.

The child also identifies with those caretakers (i.e. assumes their personality characteristics as part of the child's own developing personality). So how caretakers deal with their own frustration plays a role in the formation of the child ego (sense of self) and its level of strength.

Finally, the reactions of caretakers to the child's anxieties, disappointments and failures is crucial in the formation of the child's ego-strength. For example, one of my friends has described his parents as investing a lot of time and interest in him. He experienced them as supportive whether he succeeded or failed. He sensed they expected him to do well at things, but in a way that seemed like faith not pressure. He is a successful and happy man who I see as more of a risk-taker than most people. But he invests himself (and his money) judiciously.

On the other hand, one of my patients described how her parents 'expected me to be the best at everything I tried.' She felt they would reject her if she 'failed'. Though she was her high school valedictorian, 'married well' and is 'able to charm everyone', she has experienced life-threatening anorexia, chronic depression and is very critical of herself. In our therapy she panics when she discovers any flaw in herself. She has difficulty fully investing herself in social and vocational endeavors as well.

As a physician in training, you will certainly be criticized by senior medical staff. It's important to accept what is true about any criticism and to explicitly acknowledge it. But it's equally important to avoid overgeneralizing and overpersonalizing the criticism. For example, criticism about hurting a patient in drawing blood does not mean that you never draw blood properly or that you are insensitive.

THE ENHANCEMENT OF EGO-STRENGTH

Inherent in every difficult circumstance is an opportunity for growth. How you handle failure not only provides a clue into your character, but it is also one of the unique times as an adult that you can raise your level of ego-strength.

Failure: a chance for growth

All successful people have failed. Most chief executive officers of large corporations have been fired at least once from a job. Many people believe that the ability to motivate oneself and learn from failure are major components of a successful personality. The successful response to failure may act as the impetus for future success. A good example is Lee Iacocca who was fired from the Ford Motor Company and became the savior of the Chrysler Corporation. What may have been his greatest failure was the catalyst for one of the greatest achievements in modern corporate history. The time of failure may be one of danger, but it is also a great opportunity to enhance your ego-strength.

Effective management of difficulties

Of course it is also possible for the reverse to occur. For example, if when faced with some of the overwhelming demands of residency, you start relying upon alcohol to cope, you do so at the cost of decreasing your capacity to deal with discomfort in the future in a subtle yet predictable way. On the other hand, you may expand your coping repertoire more constructively as Dr R., a young radiologist, told me he did during his residency. He said that the personal and marital crises he experienced during residency led to his seeking psychotherapy for the first time in his life. He said it helped him deal more effectively with difficulties since that time; for example, being able to let people know he did not know the answer and ask questions, as well as to acknowledge his mistakes. He generally became more aware and accepting of himself.

Nonetheless, he, like other doctors, told me that he tended not to divulge his personal problems to fellow residents for fear of his professional image being tarnished. Fortunately for Dr R., he found another benefit from psychotherapy His image of himself as being someone who could handle a situation when things got tough was preserved because he was flexible enough to broaden his definition of what tough means.

BROAD GOALS
In her book *Pathfinders*[1], Gail Sheehy reports that people who have narrow life goals (e.g. aspire to become very wealthy, score significantly lower on life satisfaction scales than those with broad goals; see Chapter 4 on *Time Management*). Her study shows that people who score high on a sense of well-being have realistic, fluid and broad goals.

A balanced life
Residency may prove to be a great threat to your ability to lead such a balanced life. For example, Dr R. told me that he devoted so much time to his hospital work and residency that his relationship with his wife withered and ultimately died from lack of attention. This is a common occurrence in residency. Furthermore, his usual ways of relieving stress, seeing friends and routinely playing sports, were dropped because of work demands. He was ultimately able to rebalance his life through psychotherapy.

Broadening your goals
One way to broaden a goal is to focus on the process rather than simply the outcome. For example, instead of defining your goal as 'passing my boards on the first try,' your goal could be to study daily for 2 hours for the next 4 months and to take the board preparatory course. The second goal is specific, achievable and optimizes your chances to obtain your longer term outcome goal. In addition to the satisfaction inherent in such effort, it is helpful to build in some reinforcement at regular intervals, such as rewarding yourself after each daily study period with something you enjoy.

Deriving satisfaction from achievements
After achieving a long sought after goal, it is natural to experience some letdown after the initial satisfaction. It may take a while for new goals to evolve. However, some people are chronically unable to derive real satisfaction from achievements. Dr A. began seeing me in psychotherapy because of his chronic self-doubt and depression. As is true of most people, he saw these difficulties as due to problems in his current life (e.g. the stress of residency and particularly problems with his hospital supervisors). After further exploration, he saw that these problems were part of a pattern which began in his childhood. He felt his father was distant, withholding emotionally and driven, and reported his

alcoholic mother as unsupportive and critical. He also seemed to have identified with what we later came to believe was each parent's sense of inadequacy.

Like his father, the main way he tried to deal with his inadequacy feelings was to become an overachiever. However, each time he succeeded at something, he derogated his accomplishment and convinced himself that he would only feel worthwhile if he achieved more. For example, when he was accepted into a first rate medical school he began questioning its standing and wished he had applied to even more prestigious programs.

After we worked together for a couple months, Dr A. realized he was re-enacting his parents' tendency to discount his successes and expect more. Eventually, he was able to consistently catch his own tendency to dismiss his accomplishments, and was able to experience satisfaction and the ego-enhancing effects of his successes. He exhibited several of the more common reasons people can have difficulty enjoying success. For example, he used success to compensate for his deficient sense of self, while investing little in personal relationships and enjoyment. He focused upon the expectations of others in setting his goals and on their reactions to his efforts. Therefore, he derived little meaning and personal satisfaction from his successes.

Success anxiety
Another block to the ability to succeed and/or enjoy it, is success phobia or success anxiety, where achievement has become unconsciously equated with the loss of love or with punishment and retaliation. Usually this occurs because caretakers are perceived as threatened somehow by their dependant's success. The child perceives them in a way that is very uncomfortable and threatening to him- or herself. The most common pattern is for the child to feel that the same-sex parent is reacting negatively to the child's success, or at least having strong mixed feelings about such success (i.e. unresolved Oedipal feelings).

STRESS REDUCTION BASICS
This may all sound complicated and frightening, but unless you experience chronic problems in adjusting to residency, there is no need to be concerned about it. There are some basic health measures to keep in mind, however, such as remembering to regulate your diet and get as

much rest as you can, though sleep is certainly one necessity over which you will lose some control (see Chapter 6).

Regular exercise

Getting regular exercise to the extent your schedule allows it is important. Aerobic exercise is not only most helpful in terms of cardiovascular benefit, but in reducing stress as well[2].

Meditation

For more sedentary people, meditation may be a useful substitute for aerobic exercise. It also may be more feasible given schedule constraints, since it only takes 15 minutes and does not require a shower afterward. In his book, *The Relaxation Response*[3], Herbert Benson MD, described a simple and yet very effective meditation approach. He suggests that you get in a comfortable position, typically seated upright, with eyes closed. An environment free of distractions is best. Then a 'mental device', commonly called a 'mantra' which means tool for thought, is used as a focus. Each time you exhale, you say a word that has neutral meaning (e.g. word 'one'). This is continued for 10–20 minutes. Afterwards, you sit quietly for several minutes, first with eyes closed and later opened. Dr Benson and others who teach such forms of concentration meditation emphasize the need for a passive attitude, that is, calmly returning to the word 'one', or any other neutral word such as 'om', 'zarim', etc., when your mind wanders.

He presents medical research supporting the stress reduction efficacy of such regular mantra type meditation.

In contrast to concentration meditation, insight meditation is often associated with religious contemplation. Such religious meditation is also very helpful in relieving stress if you are a believer. In fact, in his most recent book, *Your Maximum Mind*[4], Herbert Benson describes how you can integrate mantra-type meditation with spiritual beliefs and contemplation.

Finally, given that you may only have a minute or two at times to replenish your psychic reserves, there are a number of excellent books of brief meditations such as the *Hazeldon Meditation Series*, as well as various religious meditation books.

The following quote is a selection from one of that series entitled *Today's Gift*[5] which has a different meditation for each date of the year:

'June 12 — The more a diamond is cut the more it sparkles (Anonymous).

There is something of value to be found even in the worst of things. Consider the oyster. When a grain of sand penetrates an oyster's shell, it irritates the oyster, making it uncomfortable. The oyster relieves the pain by coating the sand with a soothing liquid. When this liquid hardens, a pearl is formed. The very process that healed the oyster created a precious jewel for others to cherish and admire.

The way in which we deal with our own frustrations — painful though they may be — can make a difference. Pearls can be formed from our experiences, making us wiser and stronger, or grains of sand — anger, bitterness, resentment — can remain imbedded inside us. The choice is ours.'

HOW CAN I TURN MY IRRITATIONS INTO PEARLS TODAY?

Talking about it
Of course, the mainstay of coping with stress in residency is to take some reasonable risk to regularly vent your upset to someone you trust, your spouse or friend, co-worker or supervisor — anyone with whom you feel comfortable in terms of their understanding, acceptance and keeping a confidence if needed.

Approach to relaxation
Working with such serious and often life and death matters for so much of your time, can create a tendency to generalize that feeling. It is easy to feel serious and to approach leisure activities and relationships in a work-like manner. To the extent you can play tennis for the fun of it instead of trying to maintain your competitive edge, it helps. Non-competitive games such as frisbee may be especially relaxing[6]. It can help to build in leisure time instead of passively allowing work to consume all your time and attention. Introducing playfulness into your working relationships helps as well.

Accepting the inherent difficulties
It is important to face the reality that you will be placed in situations at times where you have little control and yet great responsibility. This combination is highly stressful. The introduction to the best selling book *The Road Less Traveled*[7] by psychiatrist M. Scott Peck applies.

'Life is difficult.

This is a great truth, one of the greatest truths...once we truly see this truth, we transcend it. Once we truly know that life is difficult — once we truly understand and accept that fact — the life is no longer difficult. Because once it is accepted the fact that life is difficult no longer matters.'

And so, once you truly accept the difficulties inherent in residency, you can use those irritations to create the pearls of personal and professional growth.

REFERENCES
1. Sheehy, G. (1982). *Pathfinders,* p. 625. (New York: Bantam Books)
2. Cooper, K. (1970). *The New Aerobics.* (New York: Bantam Books)
3. Benson, H. (1975). *The Relaxation Response,* p. 150. (New York: William Morrow and Co.)
4. Benson, H. (1987). *Your Maximum Mind.* (New York: Random House Inc.)
5. Anonymous (1985). *Today's Gift.* (Center City, MN: Hazeldon Educational Materials)
6. Fluegelnian, A. (1976). *New Games Book.* (New York: Doubleday Company)
7. Scott Peek, M. (1978). *The Road Less Traveled.* (New York: Simon and Shuster)

8

Intimate relationships in residency

G. Bagale

INTRODUCTION
American marriage and family life is undergoing a dramatic change. Cohabitation without marriage, marriage without children and openly gay relationships are commonplace. Women have reliable birth control and are working outside the home in increasing numbers. As a young physician, you are part of these social phenomena, but have the additional challenge of a physically and emotionally strenuous career. Furthermore, you may have a spouse who is also pursuing educational or career goals, including medicine. These choices and challenges may complicate the maintenance of an intimate relationship. While there is no sound evidence that physicians' marriages are less satisfying or more prone to divorce than average[1,2], you certainly want to maximize your relationship with your partner. This chapter will discuss forming intimate relationships and make suggestions for nurturing a healthy relationship with your significant other.

MATURING AND MATING
The majority of physicians enter residency in young adulthood, the stage of the family life cycle when developmental tasks include identity consolidation, establishing a committed relationship and launching a career[3].

Know yourself
The consolidation of your identity is crucial in developing the maturity necessary for healthy intimate relationships. Knowing yourself as an

individual person, including what matters to you in a relationship, and what you have to offer to another person, is an essential prerequisite for building a good relationship. Recognizing your own strengths and weaknesses helps you to accept both admired qualities and the inevitable weaknesses of your prospective mate.

Know what you want
Knowing what you want, and what you can live with in a relationship, will help you determine if your potential mate is acceptable the way he or she is. The courtship period provides the opportunity to live through experiences to determine your compatibility for a lifetime commitment. You will probably be disappointed if you marry with the hope or expectation that your mate's attitudes or behaviors will change after the vows are taken.

Compatibility
Although people often seek out an ideal marriage partner, successful marriages are the result of a compatible match of the two people involved. Just as there are numerous individual personalities, there are many kinds of happy marriages. A happy marriage involves the definition of mutually agreed upon lifestyles and goals. In their study of marital adjustment of resident physicians, Spendlove and colleagues found that the most important factors in marital adjustment were the perceived level of emotional support for a career and the level of such support given to the spouse for his or her career[2]. If two careers are involved, can each one accommodate the other? Can you negotiate agreements regarding educational goals, residential location, financial concerns, having children and managing the household on a day-to-day basis? Many resident households experience considerable strain if both people are working. There is greater relationship stress for residents with working spouses if household chores are not shared[4].

Influence of families
Marriages exist within a sociocultural context which influences the expectations of both partners. The most immediate influences come from the families of the couple. Although predictions cannot be made with total accuracy about the effects of family on an individual or marriage, generally speaking, most people live their lives in a similar or opposite fashion to that of their parents. Major life decisions, such as where to

live, career choices and childrearing are influenced by the individual's emotional interconnections and reactions to the previous generation. For the most part, the greater the emotional impact of family experiences on the individual, the greater the likelihood that this will influence choices in adult intimate relationships. Here again, individuals need to have consolidated their own identities in order to establish a successful relationship within the context of their extended families. The individual who is enmeshed in his or her family cannot commit adequately to a relationship outside the family. On the other hand, the individual who is emotionally cut-off from the family due to unresolved conflicts will probably experience relationship problems traceable to these conflicts. For example, one young couple had difficulty coping with the resident's spending more time away from home than necessary. The resident had coped with his critical parents by cutting off contact with them. When his wife criticized his time away, he began to withdraw from her, spending more time at the hospital.

Importance of a successful relationship

Your success in establishing a healthy intimate relationship has ramifications for future stages in your family life cycle. The patterns of interaction you establish now will probably become characteristic of your marital and family relationships in the future. As a resident, you are highly motivated and perfectionistic, characteristics which serve you well in acquiring professional knowledge. However, you also need to develop yourself personally, including your relationship with your mate. Beware of the tendency to put things off until the end of residency. Some things can be put on hold, but a pattern of neglect in a relationship can easily continue with the lifelong demands of your profession, resulting in covert marital discord[5].

GENERAL TIPS FOR A SUCCESSFUL RELATIONSHIP

Although much has been written regarding the stresses of residency on intimate relationships, residents and their mates have told me they did not fully comprehend the impact of residency training on their lives until they lived through it. Resident couples cope with the consequences of long hours and days apart, as well as unpredicted interruptions in time together. When there is time together, residents often have depleted their physical and emotional energy, resulting in disappointment for both. In *Married to their Careers*, Gerber quotes a second year resident:

'When I come home, especially after I've been on-call the night before, I just want to pour myself into bed. A lot of times I'm not even hungry. When I am, I'd almost like somebody to feed it to me. I know it's not fair to Ellen, but I don't want to talk to her. I don't have the energy to talk to anyone...and sex? Forget it. Last week she started to get undressed and I fell asleep...Doctors are really sexy, huh?[6]'

Additionally, the gratification residents experience in learning medicine in the hospital environment can leave a partner feeling left out or in competition for time and attention.

The challenges of finding time and energy to sustain an intimate relationship between two residents are likely to be greater than those with one resident. At the same time, in a two-resident couple, both partners understand the immersion and gratification of residency training. Also, each has invested in becoming a physician, an individually rewarding and mutually valued professional goal. (See Table 8-1.)

Value of the relationship
Given the demands of residency, how do you nurture a healthy relationship with a mate? First of all, realize that your relationship is important enough to warrant attention while you are a resident. The relationship patterns you establish now will probably become characteristic of your future together. Your relationship with your mate is your main source of coping with the stresses of being a physician, but it is often the first and most neglected aspect of a physician's life when other demands become pressing[5].

Communication
Find the time to talk, talk, talk. Take at least 15 minutes a day to discuss concerns, feelings, activities, plans, whatever is important to either of you. Talking time must be carved out of busy schedules and jealously protected. Even resident couples on call can find 15 minutes for a phone conversation. Better yet, dinner together at the hospital, whether you settle for hospital fare, pack a picnic, or share a carry-out pizza, can give you the precious time your relationship needs.

Learn to be direct and explicit in expressing your needs and feelings to each other. Talk about the embarrassing or threatening topics, or they will fester under the surface of your relationship. Try to express feelings such as anger, hurt, and embarrassment by letting your mate know that this is what you feel — 'I feel' messages — rather than blaming or critical ones.

Table 8-1. Resource organizations

American Association of Physicians for Human Rights,
273 Church Street, San Francisco, California 94114, USA.
(Tel: 415-255-4547.)

American Medical Association Auxiliary Inc,
535 North Dearborn Street, Chicago, Illinois 60610, USA.
(Tel: 312-645-5000.)

Whether or not you agree with your mate, listen to and acknowledge that this is how he or she feels. If you can validate each other's feelings in this way, your relationship will become an emotionally safe place. On the other hand, demeaning, humiliating or vengeful responses to an honest expression of feelings serve no constructive purpose in resolving your differences, and may harm your relationship far beyond the issue at hand. If a disagreement begins to deteriorate into this destructive mode of communication, either partner should call a time-out for each person to regain control of his or her feelings. Usually, within 30 minutes to an hour, the partners should be cooled off enough to resume communicating. Ideally, the partner who called the time-out should take the initiative in restarting the discussion (S. Fabick, unpublished). A final word about talking: for every negative thing expressed to your mate, say five positive things. Observe yourself for the next few days, and see if you are maintaining this 1:5 ratio.

Develop the fine art of negotiation and compromise. No two people completely agree all the time. In a healthy relationship, the goal is to find workable (not necessarily perfect) solutions in resolving differences. Work on being flexible and collaborative in solving problems, rather than adopting a win/lose stance with your mate over differences. For residents, who spend the majority of their time gathering and making decisions based on facts and logic, it can be a real challenge to shift into a collaborative stance which takes into account feelings, opinions and emotional needs. While it is a good idea to establish some general ground rules for day-to-day operations, allow for the possibility that these may change over time, and may need to be renegotiated. After a couple months, you may find that you would rather cook than wash the dishes, which may suit your neatnik mate just fine!

Importance of a social network

Keep active with friends and family. If you relocate to a different area, it may require additional effort to develop new social networks, but it is worth the effort for your mental well-being. Due to their common interests in medicine and limited leisure time, residents and their partners most often socialize together, which can be an excellent network for recreation and social support. Cultivating other relationships which may evolve naturally in your social milieu (e.g. church, neighborhood or partner's workplace) broadens your experiences and your support systems.

The task of developing a social network is more difficult, but is critical for gay and lesbian couples. Due to the uncertainty of acceptance and the fear of adverse professional consequences if you reveal your sexual orientation, you often find yourself in a dilemma over how 'out of the closet' you want to be, and with whom to socialize as a couple. Many gay physicians keep a low profile in their first year of residency, until they determine how out they want to be. If you do not have a social network, there is increased pressure on your relationship, as you and your partner must rely on each other to meet your emotional needs. Since your time for social contact is limited, gay physicians advise that you seek out other gay or lesbian couples more actively than straight friends. Sometimes tough choices over whether to spend precious time over holidays with your partner or your family of origin, who do not accept your partner, must be made. Try to negotiate compromises with all your loved ones, but if this is not possible, do not leave your partner alone. The American Association of Physicians for Human Rights is a good resource for information for gay and lesbian physicians (see Table 8-1).

HAVING CHILDREN

Since the time period for residency training coincides with the ages at which most people in our society begin raising their families, you and your mate may find yourselves making decisions regarding whether to move into this next stage of the family life cycle. Modern advances in birth control and reproductive medicine provide you with reliable family planning options, whether you decide to have child(ren) during residency, defer this until later, or not have children at all. Generally, it is advisable to allow about a year to effect the transition into a committed relationship before having children. From a system of two adults who can function independently, a child adds another person to the family who is dependent on these adults. Both you and your mate should carefully consider the responsibilities of raising a child. While it may take considerable time and deliberation to decide when and how to raise your children, these are some of the most important decisions you will make in your life, and they should not be treated lightly.

Include the following in your decision-making:

(1) *Children require 24-hour a day care!* How much quality time will each of you have with your child? With one or both of you having responsibilities outside the home, how will you provide the nurturance and care you want for your child? Are there extended family members who can help in the care of your child? What other options for child care are available, daily, occasionally, or on an emergency basis? Having your child with caretakers that you trust is essential, both for your child's sake and your own peace of mind. Worrying about your child's welfare when you are at work is distracting and emotionally stressful. If you are a woman resident, be aware that you may experience guilt or ambivalence over the limitations that residency places on your relationship with your child, even under the best of circumstances. There are no established predictors for these feelings, so give considerable thought to how you would cope, if this should happen to you.

(2) *What are the parental leave policies of your program and your mate's employment?* Women residents, in particular, should consider the physical demands of a pregnancy, the amount of time off allowed for having a baby, how that may affect their progress in their residency, and the attitudes of faculty and other residents regarding pregnancy and time away from the program. In general, women who have become pregnant in residency indicate they would prefer to wait until after their first year of training before conceiving. In one survey, 70% of women physicians considered the completion of residency to be the best time to become pregnant[7].

(3) *Is adequate housing for a family with children available?* Is it within reasonable proximity to your training program, your mate's employment or school, family, and childcare? Can you afford it?

A WORD TO THE SIGNIFICANT OTHER

You have entered into a relationship which can be both rewarding and challenging. The noble mission of the medical profession, the financial security, and the respected social status of the physician family will be a part of your lives, along with the ramifications of living with someone who must routinely confront the most intense of human experiences.

Independence
It is important that you develop an independent life and satisfying activities of your own, in addition to your relationship with your resident partner. Be a homemaker, a parent, a community volunteer, pursue your own career, or all of these.

Effort
During your partner's residency training, you may devote considerable effort to keep your relationship viable. Do not keep a scorecard of who is giving more. Your partner will probably lose, but you will just win a pile of resentment. Work at being patient with the unavoidable. It is normal to be upset when your partner misses your boss's dinner party due to an emergency with a patient — but you eventually have to let it go, or your relationship will not survive. Take the initiative and be creative in planning some fun together, whether it is a love letter stuck in a pocket or a picnic on your day off. One resident once told me that the best thing his partner did for him during his residency was to 'kidnap' him for an occasional weekend to a motel away from the hospital, the kids, everything.

Healthy lifestyle
Residents are notoriously poor at maintaining a healthy lifestyle. They often eat whatever is readily available and get little, if any, exercise. Develop a healthy diet. Exercising moderately a few times a week has the obvious physical benefits, and is correlated with reduced stress in intimate relationships of residents[4].

The American Medical Association Auxiliary is a good resource for information on supporting physician marriages (see Table 8-1).

CONCLUSIONS
Developing an intimate relationship which can nurture the partners and withstand the pressures and rapid changes of modern society is a challenge for people entering medicine in the 1990s. You need to have a good sense of your own identity and accept that you both have weaknesses as well as strengths. Establish mutual and independent life goals that are in concordance with each other. Cultivate and maintain your

skills in communicating and negotiating compromises. Try to be patient and flexible with each other. Keep in touch with family, friends, and those meaningful relationships that enrich your lives, and be open to new people and experiences. Your relationship is between two human beings; one or both of you happens to be a physician!

ACKNOWLEDGEMENTS

The author is grateful to the many physicians who shared their residency experiences with her, especially Dr James Boyd, Dr Steve Hartleib and Dr JoAnn Kaplan.

REFERENCES

1. Doherty, W. and Burge, S. (1989). Divorce among physicians, comparisons with other occupational groups. *J. Am. Med. Assoc.*, **261**, 2374-7
2. Spendlove, D., Reed, B., Whitman, N., Slattery, M., French, T. and Horwood, K. (1990). Marital adjustment among housestaff and new attorneys. *Acad. Med.*, **65**, 599-603
3. Carter, E. and McGoldrick, M. (eds.) (1980). *The Changing Family Life Cycle: A Framework for Family Therapy.* (New York: Gardner Press)
4. Landau, C., Hall, S., Wartman, S. and Macko, M. (1986). Stress in social and family relationships during the medical residency. *J. Med. Educ.*, **61**, 654-60
5. Gabbard, G. and Menninger, R. (1989). The psychology of postponement in the medical marriage. *J. Am. Med. Assoc.*, **261**, 2378-81
6. Gerber, L. (1983). *Married to Their Careers: Career and Family Dilemmas in Doctor's Lives.* (New York: Tavistock)
7. Sinal, S., Weavil, P. and Camp, M. (1988). Survey of women physicians on issues relating to pregnancy during a medical career. *J. Med. Educ.*, **63**, 531-8

FURTHER READING

1. Howell, J. and Schroeder, D. (1984). *Physician Stress: A Handbook for Coping.* (Baltimore: University Park Press)
2. Phelan, S. (1988). Pregnancy during residency I. The decision 'to be or not to be'. *Obstet. Gynecol.*, **72**, 425-31
3. Shem, S. (1988). *The House of God.* (New York: Dell)
4. Van Buren, K. (1988). How to survive your husband's residency. *Resident and Staff Physician*, **35**, 84-9

9

Women in medicine: the balancing act

M. B. Riba

INTRODUCTION

Women students and house officers have difficulties in a profession that has traditionally been the province of men[1]. Often, the focus of tension is on maintaining a career while having a personal life outside of medicine. There are a host of pressures that fall particularly on the shoulders of women trainees. This chapter will identify some of these difficulties and offer strategies or ideas for tackling the juggling many of you will be doing in the months and years ahead.

THE TRANSITION FROM STUDENT TO HOUSE OFFICER

About 40% of the current medical students in this country are women[2]. As more women enter the profession, both opportunities and challenges present themselves. One must decide, for example, what specialty of medicine will offer the most controllable lifestyle choice.

Deciding on which specialty

Are the challenges and excitement of going into general surgery conducive to your plans for marriage and child-rearing or would a subspecialty in surgery, such as ophthalmology, offer more flexibility? When deciding, it is often helpful to speak to women mentors or those who have crossed this path before. Acknowledging that choosing a specialty is difficult is often the first step in solving the problem. Of course the real dilemma is that we cannot foretell the future but are being asked to make decisions that will have a long-term impact. Who would not be anxious, worried and uptight? Most of us just end up making a best guess, based on clerkship and elective experiences in medical schools, advice from mentors and advisers, etc., and wishes and goals for our personal lives. There are many residents, women and men, who retrain or modify their practices later if their original decisions do not work out. Choosing a career is not cast in stone for either gender.

Personal relationships

The process of actually graduating from medical school, saying goodbye to fellow students, friends and family in the community, perhaps moving to a city far away, finding new lodging, new supports, etc., are difficult and troubling transitional issues that women must face. Often a decision must be made on how to end or change relationships with significant others because of the impending shift to becoming a house officer. The literature suggests that, compared to law students, female medical students end personal relationships sooner due to the stress of training[3]. These changes can be premature or poorly time based on the development of the relationship, but necessary because of the schedule in the course of training. There are some women who choose to use the time between graduation and beginning house staff training to get married, take a honeymoon, etc., and so may be starting the residency years as part of a newly married couple with all those inherent changes.

Whatever the specifics, you will no doubt be beginning the residency with new issues regarding your personal life that will impact on your professional development. Recognizing that this is normal, that there will be anxieties as there always are with transitions may help to underscore the normalcy of the problem(s).

Support programs

What are some other coping strategies? Many medical schools and residency programs provide opportunities for peer groups to meet and prepare for and work through the transition. The groups can become a nidus for support, education and encouragement about what lies ahead, as well as offering problem solving and coping strategies. Often, women physicians on the faculty or in the community present what their experience has shown them in their own balancing acts and provide advice. If there are not such groups in your program, there may be women on the faculty who would be willing to help sponsor such a project, or at least help get it started. Organizations such as the American Medical Women's Association

(AMWA), Alexandria, Virginia, 703-838-0500, and specialty organizations (American Psychiatric Association, Washington DC, 202-682-6000; American Medical Association, Chicago, Illinois, 312-464-5000) have local groups and resources who can also help.

Some residency programs have very good orientation programs for house staff and their significant others, including children. This helps to acknowledge the hard work that lies ahead for *everyone* in the relationship and alerts family members to potential methods of averting difficulties. Husbands of residents often work much longer hours than wives of residents, and female house officers spend substantially more time on household chores than their male counterparts[4]. It especially helps couples and families to plan and co-ordinate such mundane efforts as meal planning, child-care arrangements, and tasks like who will be doing the laundry or putting out the trash when on-call, which is especially difficult.

THE BIOLOGICAL CLOCK

A survey by Revinson *et al.*[5] of 558 women physicians in academic medicine showed that the academic clock competes with the biological clock and may even tick more loudly[5]. When the women were asked about family size and what they would change if they could, one-third said they would have had more children. On average, women physicians were 31 years old when their first child was born compared with an average age of 23 for women in the general population. This delay in childbearing points to the dilemma faced by women who must make career choices against the backdrop of a ticking biological clock. In Dr Levinson's study, 80% of the women who were married had a child, but very rarely before beginning medical school. One-fourth of them had their children during residency, but almost one-half had them after all their formal training, including fellowship. Many of these women did not take any time off before the delivery; and on average, only took 6 weeks off after the delivery before returning to full-time work. More than one-half of the women, in retrospect, felt that this was too short a time.

Pregnancy during residency

Outcome. Klebanoff *et al.* studied the outcomes of pregnancy during residency for 4412 women using a national questionnaire[6]. Results of the survey indicated that in spite of working longer hours, working later into their pregnancies, and working with reportedly less supportive co-workers and supervisors, women residents have a risk of adverse pregnancy outcome that is similar to that for the wives of male residents. However, women residents who work more than 100 hours per week (15% during the first trimester, decreasing to 8% during the third) may be at increased risk for preterm delivery. There have been other studies which have reported that pregnant physicians do have an increased risk of intrauterine growth retardation, placental abruption and pregnancy-induced hypertension.

Problems encountered. Breast feeding, child-care arrangements, keeping up with training requirements, dealing with possible resentment from other house staff during pregnancy and subsequent maternity leave are just some of the multitude of issues that confront you if you should choose motherhood during residency. It was not too long ago that residents in some programs needed to get the approval from residency directors even before contemplating getting pregnant so that coverage could be planned! Even today, there are many programs where maternity leave is deducted from the vacation allowance or where there is no paid maternity leave. Many teaching hospitals do not even grant maternity leave[7]. Most residency programs have no specific policies regarding maternity leave [8,9]. Since maternity, paternity and family leave affect all residents, I would strongly advise residents to use this issue as a major selection criterion for choosing and staying with a training program.

The pressures of dealing with the ticking biological clock while attempting to get through the residency are difficult indeed. Having a child in the early years of a residency when there are a great many on-call responsibilities and the rotations are more grueling and intensive can be very trying. The resident who is pregnant and takes leave is subject to criticism or anger by unsympathetic colleagues (men and women). She may worry about the gap in her training and her abilities to be a 'good mother', a 'good physician' and a 'good wife,' etc. Finally, the question of the value of a physician–mother's time at home during an infant's first months is a more difficult problem and one not as yet addressed in most sectors of residency training.

Know your program's policies. Knowing the maternity and paternity leave policies before starting a residency is very helpful. Understanding how the coverage occurs for your fellow house staff can not only help deal with their feelings and work load problems, but may impact on you if others in your program become pregnant. These policies should be in writing. Furthermore, you need to find out the consequences if you must take more time off than it states in the policy. Will the residency program guarantee to hold your job? Can the didactics and training sequences be provided within reason upon your return or will you need to wait? Will not only your job but a stipend be guaranteed if your maternity leave is lengthy? Will someone arrange to cover your on-call duties or will that be left up to you? Will you need to make up the on-call hours upon your return? Are there ways you can rejoin the residency program in a part-time capacity or work flexible hours? These are just a few questions you may want to explore with your training director.

Choices. Even if you choose to wait till you are finished with your training to have a child, how will this affect your career? It will also depend on the number of children you ultimately plan to have, the spacing you want between children, as well as the age when you and your husband envision becoming parents. The list goes on....

My first daughter was four when I started medical school. Eight years later, at the age of 39 when I was a fourth-year resident in psychiatry, we had our second daughter (same husband). The spacing was not exactly ideal, but I just could not have coped earlier in medical school or residency with having an infant, an active older child, and a physician–husband who also worked long hours. At the same time, my biological clock was ticking away and my husband (and I, unfortunately) were not getting any younger.

No easy answers. It takes some planning and realization that there are no right or wrong solutions or blueprints that will fit all of our situations. Knowing your program's policies in advance regarding the questions above may help you in your decision-making process. In addition, advocating for day-care availability in hospitals, support groups where residents can openly discuss problems concerning conflicts which may arise, and identifying women role models would also be other ways to improve the situation[10].

SEXUAL HARASSMENT AND SEXUAL DISCRIMINATION
Sexual harassment and discrimination are national issues that are receiving more attention in medical training and academics. This was exemplified by the problems Dr Frances Conley faced in her career as a Stanford neurosurgeon[11], when she was passed over for academic advancement because of her gender.

Impact on women

Although there are few data regarding the actual impact of these issues on women residents, surveys suggest that women medical students and residents are more likely than men to have been physically or sexually harassed, and that women's harassers are of higher professional stature[12].

When harassed or discriminated against, women experience it as a hostile environment for training and one that, at a minimum, interferes with work performance. These experiences often go unreported because women do not feel confident that they will be helped[12]. Women sometimes have difficulty telling their significant others about harassment for fear that it will be construed as if she were 'flirting' or 'coming on' to the harasser.

Harassment and discrimination affect your self-esteem, are demoralizing and degrading, and impair trust towards colleagues and superiors if they are allowed to persist within a training environment. Trainees' education suffers, as does patient care. A career in academic medicine certainly would not be chosen. On the contrary, a trainee would most likely leave a hostile environment as soon as possible since the top echelon in an academic institution sets the tone for the educational setting[13].

What action can be taken?

The legal approach is one avenue for recourse. Training programs should have a method of responding to formal complaints of harassment and discrimination when they occur. Prevention is the key. The residency and/or institution must have in place a visible means to monitor these issues and provide education and training. Finally, women trainees need to be taught to recognize behavior they should not have to tolerate, learn prompt responses when the unwelcome behavior occurs, and to seek help[12].

ROLE STRAIN

'Role strain' is an umbrella heading for understanding and coping with the many hats women residents wear and the stress that results.

The causes

Residents, male and female, experience stress when their preconceived notion of the role and lifestyles of physicians clashes with their own busy, difficult lives. This may be magnified when watching peers in other professions become financially secure sooner or have easier lifestyles.

Women residents, in particular, may become more anxious about their spouses, children and parents and are more likely to become depressed when hospital responsibilities interfere with child care[14,15]. In a number of studies of women junior house officers, stress and depression were related to overwork, feelings of being overwhelmed and overloaded, as well as worrying about the impact of the job and career on personal life[16]. Time pressures and feelings that you have to be in several places at once create escalating feelings of anxiety and low self-esteem.

Within training programs, women residents may have fewer social supports than men[17] and may feel excluded from the fraternity of male peers. Women residents may perceive prejudice from patients, sexual harassment at work, a lack of female role models and discrimination by senior doctors[16]. Another role strain is that women residents must sometimes cope with spouses who are jealous of their success. If you come home and talk about something that you did well at work, it may be viewed as boastful. On the other hand, if you do not discuss it, you may be holding back on sharing some of your successes and part of your day's activities with your spouse. Behavior that may be viewed as 'assertive' in male residents may be labeled as 'aggressive' in female residents[15]. It sometimes is difficult to turn off the persona you have at the hospital, especially when you are fatigued and spent. The dilemma is sometimes giving so much emotional and physical energy at the job that there is little left for your family, let alone yourself.

Feeling pulled in different directions adds to the general worries women and men residents have about such diverse issues as their competencies as physicians, future employability, worries about contracting diseases from patients, financial burdens and sleep deprivation.

The toll. In women residents this can be quite high. In a group of family medicine residents, women experienced a higher incidence and greater severity of personal or emotional problems than men. These problems were associated with an increased percentage of women who had used alcohol during the preceding year, had used alcohol daily, had increased use of alcohol over the 2 years before the survey, and had had perceptions of being overweight and were on calorie-restricted diets[18]. Anxiety and depression are common among residents with women at greater risk of depression during internship than men[19]. Among female physicians, the rate of suicide is highest among young and single women[20]. Performance at work may be impaired because of anxiety and depression. Marital problems negatively impact on residents' performance[21]. Male and female residents are concerned that their current relationships will not survive the stresses of residency[17].

What strategies reduce role strain?

I sometimes find it helpful to view such problems in this way: what do I have control over and what is out of my control? Another way to phrase this is: what is fixable and what is not? It helps me if I can at least get to the point of understanding that the problems exist, what corrective actions should be taken, and then figuring out if the solution or action comes under my control in any way. A fair amount of anxiety comes off my shoulders when I realize that there is a problem but there is no way I can personally fix it right now.

Whatever strategy works for you, it usually involves some cognitive work such as assessment and recognition of the problem and then a process by which remedies are reviewed and responsibilities to individuals or groups are placed.

The major problem with being a woman house officer is trying to solve problems while feeling fatigued, sleep deprived, overworked, overloaded and guilty of not being able to 'do it all.' For many women who have worked and studied for years to get to the point of being a house officer, it becomes confusing why she may feel depressed and anxious, etc. The good news is that internship is the most difficult year and it does get better. The idea is to minimize personal catastrophes and to begin to think of at least some ways of enjoying yourself while a house officer.

Finally, psychotherapy, either individual, group or couples can be extremely useful, effective and efficient in the long run. Many female residents I see worry about the time off from the job, possible stigma, and what the meaning is of needing psychotherapy, etc. Most good residency training directors understand the strains and pulls on residents and so can assist you in getting the help you need and provide the names of therapists experienced in working with trainees. Many programs in fact encourage residents to seek psychotherapy sooner rather than later and have arrangements with psychiatry clinics or student mental health services to give residents care in a confidential setting and often at reduced rates.

The suggestion list is long and you will probably only have time to consider a few of these (maybe just one!). Assessing who your supports are, family or friends, would be a good starting point. Let them know what may be helpful to you. This could be picking up take-out food once a week and meeting you at your apartment. Make plans to spend your next day off together and ask them to organize it. Ask a friend to watch your child so that you can go out with your spouse. Ask a parent to come and stay for a few days to provide emotional support.

Sometimes there are senior house officers who know some time-saving ways to get you out of the hospital earlier. You may find, for example, that getting into work earlier (groan) will save you a lot more time later in the day, etc.

Additionally, there are other chapters in this handbook that address some of the difficulties house officers must handle. The chapters on 'Time Management,' 'Sleep and Shift Work,' 'Starting a New Job,' and 'Emotional Survival in Residency' offer additional information on the issues addressed above.

CONCLUSIONS

How do women in medicine manage to balance career and family responsibilities? In one study by Levinson *et al.*, coping strategies were grouped into these categories: changing structural aspects of their lives, increasing efficiency, limiting personal expectations and increasing social supports[22].

Diverse, creative and personalized methods must be used to cope with the juggling that women must do when in medicine. I can tell you from personal experience that the balls do fall, the juggling act sometimes goes awry, and you may have to start again. The anticipatory anxiety is sometimes worse than the actual result.

Recognizing that there are limits to what we can do personally and professionally until our profession becomes more gender sensitive and female user-friendly may be a way to help us all in our balancing acts.

REFERENCES

1. Geis, R. E., Jesilow, P. and Geis, G. (1991). The Amelia Stern syndrome; a diagnosis of a condition among female physicians? *Soc. Sci. Med.*, **33**, 967–71

2. Reiser, L. W., Sledge, W. H., Fenton, W. and Leaf, P. (1993). Beginning careers in academic psychiatry for women — 'Bermuda Triangle'? *Am. J. Psychiatry*, **150**, 1392–7

3. Clark, E. J. and Rieker, P. P. (1986). Gender differences in relationships and stress of medical and law students. *J. Med. Educ.*, **61**, 32–40

4. Landau, C., Hall, S., Wartman, S. A. and Macko, M. B. (1986). Stress in social and family relationships during the medical residency. *J. Med. Educ.*, **61,** 654–60

5. Levinson, W., Tolle, S. W. and Lewis, C. (1989). Women in academic medicine; combining career and family. *N. Engl. J. Med.*, **321,** 1511–17

6. Klebanoff, M. A., Shiono, P. and Rhoads, G. G. (1990). Outcomes of pregnancy in a national sample of resident physicians. *N. Engl. J. Med.*, **323,** 1040-5

7. Little, A. B. (1990). Why can't a woman be more like a man? *N. Engl. J. Med.*, **323,** 1064–5

8. Sayres, M., Wyshak, G., Denterlein, G., Apfel, R., Shore, E. and Federman, D. (1986). Pregnancy during residency. *N. Engl. J. Med.*, **314,** 418–23

9. Sinal, S., Weavil, P. and Camp, M. G. (1988). Survey of women physicians on issues relating to pregnancy during a medical career. *J. Med. Educ.*, **63,** 531–8

10. Young-Shumate, L., Kramer, T. and Beresin, E. (1993). Pregnancy during graduate medical training. *Acad. Med.*, **68,** 792–9

11. Gross, J. (1991). Female surgeon's quitting touches nerve at medical schools. *N. Y. Times,* **July 14,** 10

12. Komaromy, M., Bindman, A. B., Haber, R. J. and Sande, M. A. (1993). Sexual harassment in medical training. *N. Engl. J. Med.*, **328,** 322–6

13. Conley, F. K. (1993). Toward a more perfect world — eliminating sexual discrimination in academic medicine. *N. Engl. J. Med.*, **328,** 351–2

14. Colford, J. M. and McPhee, S. J. (1989). The ravelled sleeve of care. *J. Am. Med. Assoc.*, **261,** 889–93

15. Wolfe, E. and Jones, H. (1985). Problems experienced by residents in internal medicine training. *West. J. Med.*, **42,** 570–2

16. Firth-Cozens, J. (1990). Source of stress in women junior house officers. *Br. Med. J.*, **301,** 89–91

17. Korna, L. and Litt, I. (1988). House staff well-being. *West. J. Med.*, **148,** 97–101

18. Young, E. H. (1987). Relationship of residents' emotional problems, coping behaviors, and gender. *J. Med. Educ.*, **62,** 642–50

19. Ford, C. V. and Wentz, D. K. (1984). The internship year: a study of sleep, mood states, and psychophysiologic parameters. *South. Med.*, **77,** 1435–42

20. Notman, M. T. (1975). Suicide in female physicians. *Psychiatric Opinion*, **12,** 29–30

21. Nelson, F. and Henry, W. (1978). Psychosocial factors seen as problems by family practice residents and their spouses. *J. Fam. Pract.*, **6,** 581–9

22. Levinson, W., Kaufman, K. and Tolle, S. W. (1992). Women in academic medicine; strategies for balancing career and personal life. *J. Am. Med. Wom. Assoc.*, **41,** 25–8

10

Success as an international medical graduate

K. K. Sawhney and P. E. Sawhney

INTRODUCTION

According to the American Medical Association, in 1992 there were approximately 165 000 international medical graduates (IMGs) in the US, making up approximately 22% of the entire physician work force[1]. International medical graduates are the physicians who have been educated outside of the US, its territories and Canada. They may be US-born, naturalized citizens or on a special visa. There is a long-standing history of their presence: Dr Benjamin Rush of Pennsylvania was an IMG who signed the Declaration of Independence in 1772. International medical graduates have made a very positive impact on all aspects of medicine, especially in patient care, teaching and research. A significant number of IMGs have received Nobel prizes in medicine and science. They are an integral part of the US health care system.

From the time of arrival into the US to becoming a successful, well-trained physician, the entire process can seem long, difficult and even painful at times. However, I hope to make that transition a little easier by offering the following observations and suggestions.

THE TRANSITION PROCESS (FROM FOREIGNER TO FRIEND)

At least initially, all IMGs go through a self-recognition process. At this stage, almost all feel a sense of inadequacy, rejection and incompetence, as well as social and professional isolation. These feelings are a direct result of their inability to recognize and respond to the new cultural cues. The newly arrived IMG is probably not fluent in the language nor effective in the non-verbal communication in this unfamiliar cultural environment.

For most, initial language difficulties not only impede medical training but also contribute to feelings of devaluation and lowered self-esteem. The consequence of all of this is the inability to treat their patients effectively. This problem is further compounded among those who are married, by their spouses experiencing a profound sense of social isolation and loneliness. The significant other has very distinct needs of their own and may not have a job or training program that might otherwise at least give them a sense of belonging somewhere[2,3].

International medical graduates are also faced with problems of overcoming common stereotypic images; that of being withdrawn and timid individuals, slow to learn to communicate effectively, reluctant to assume clinical responsibility and unable to perform effectively in clinical examination situations[3]. The result is that at least temporarily the IMG feels unwelcome, stressed out and inferior to his US counterparts. The important thing to remember is that these feelings can be temporary, if you recognize the source of the negative feelings you can act to overcome them.

Do not despair, for there is good news in this message. Research has shown that with the proper training in a residency program, IMGs can perform on par, and in some cases, out-perform their US counterparts in patient management as well as board examinations. Patient acceptance of well-trained IMGs is excellent[4-9]. Integration into the US system, becoming knowledgeable about cultural differences and learning to communicate effectively will all have a significant impact on the transition process.

Integration

Upon arriving in the US an IMG and his or her spouse experiences, probably for the first time, the reality of being an alien. Even among 250 million people, he or she feels lonely and alone. At first, you may be reluctant to identify with the American lifestyle, as well as having a sense of ethnic and social isolation. You will probably miss your family immensely, have feelings of professional incompetence, experience prejudice and often feel excluded professionally and socially[2,3].

It is not difficult to understand then, why IMGs tend to gravitate towards their own, forming their own small groups. This provides them with a sense of security and the approval that they are so desperately seeking. These small groups provide the reassurance they need through comparing and validating their feelings and experiences. It may further provide an important opportunity to develop a social network that is meaningful to their spouses. 'My wife did not feel comfortable with Americans', I overheard one IMG saying. 'She wanted us to have our leisure time to ourselves, among our friends from Peru, where we could talk in our own language and make our own jokes that we could all understand. But gradually she started to meet and make friends with the neighbors, and other doctor's wives, and even clerks in the grocery store. She gradually became more and more confident and now we have all kinds of American friends.' Spouses do play an important role in the construction of social contacts with Americans.

Cultural differences

International medical graduates have special difficulties because they are torn between two distinct and often very different cultures. They have long since embraced native cultural values and now must adapt to new ones in order to be accepted and effective. Everything may seem 'foreign' to the IMG upon arrival in the US. The food, dress and language are the obvious differences, but these only begin to describe the confusing and often embarrassing situations that the IMG will face. I remember an incident when I first arrived in the US. I was attending a party hosted by my senior resident. Everyone present ordered steak, so when it was my turn to order, I was afraid to order anything but steak. I did not have a clue as to what steak even was. When the waiter served this huge piece of beef dripping with blood, I made a beeline to the bathroom and deposited my stomach contents into the toilet. I had never seen such a huge piece of meat in my life.

A friend shared his memories of arrival into the US. 'I was sitting in the airport cafeteria, waiting to change planes to go to Detroit. I ordered a cup of tea. The waitress brought a little white bag with a cup of hot water. I tore the little white bag open and dumped the tea leaves into the water. When I asked the waitress for the tea strainer, she thought I was crazy. I had never seen a tea bag before!'

I have one final story to illustrate my point relating to cultural differences. 'When I arrived at Miami Airport, this man helps me with my luggage. I thought, wow! What a country. Everyone is so helpful here. I did not know you were supposed to tip the guy. He sent me to hell and back!'

Some easy and private ways to become more familiar with the American culture are to read everything you can get your hands on. This should include several different newspapers daily, magazines and professional journals. Become more knowledgeable in American history and literature. Watch television! You will pick up the American slang, humor, mannerisms, dress, customs and behavior, just to name a few. Television programming can provide a wealth of information on the American way of life. A knowledge of sports is also useful as it is an integral part of American life and will provide you with common points of discussion and casual talk during any gathering.

You do not have to change your cultural or religious beliefs in order to 'fit in.' However, you do have to participate in the American experience. If you act like a foreigner, talk like a foreigner and look like a foreigner, you will get treated like one. There are cultural training programs available in most cities. Adult education programs can give you a great place to start.

Communication: the language and accents

Another significant problem faced by the IMG is their inadequate linguistic skill. Although most may have some knowledge of formal English, they lack skill in common English usage. Besides the obvious problems that an accent presents, they have to learn the colloquialisms as well as the local humor in order to develop any facility with the language. One option is to enroll in language courses immediately upon their arrival to the US. Many hospitals provide courses in American slang for arriving IMGs. Oakwood Hospital in Dearborn, Michigan, provides accent reduction courses in their first year of training. It is imperative that the spouses of IMGs also enroll in accent reduction courses, as well as courses in English and slang. It has been demonstrated that when the IMG goes home at night, he speaks his native language with his family, thereby taking him longer to make the necessary change in his speech. Accent reduction requires constant practice. Some training programs have taken the problem of accent reduction seriously and speech pathology departments in most hospitals are equipped to work with graduate trainees in the reduction of their accents. Personally, I have seen remarkable results in many cases.

Remember that communication is a very complex process. It is a learned process. It is not just the words we speak, it involves an understanding of history, literature, behavior, expectations and sexual roles. It includes the entire spectrum of emotions. It involves the parent–child roles, that of obedience and behavior towards authority. All of the aspects of communication are fairly unique in the US.

It goes without saying that the need to communicate effectively is profound, especially for physicians.

Male/female relationships

Relationships between men and women in the workplace is a very complex topic and there are volumes of books and periodicals devoted to this subject. I will discuss a few issues that may help the new IMG in making the transition into the American workforce.

As a newly arriving male IMG, I was unprepared for the demeanor and dress of the so-called 'typical' American female. American women are typically well informed, outgoing, friendly, and they smile a lot. Professional women usually wear either dresses or suits, leaving legs, neck and upper chest exposed to some degree. At first I wondered what they wanted from me, but I gradually came to realize that this was just one of the many cultural differences that I would experience (as well as one of the first of many big blows to my ego).

In the hospital setting, it is expected that all members of the health care team, both male and female, will actively participate in the care and management of the patient. The nursing staff is very well trained and are free to give their opinions and offer suggestions on their patients' care. I hope the IMG does not feel threatened by this involvement, since the nursing staff as well as other members of the health care team can be a great source of information, support and assistance.

Sometimes, depending on the country of origin, significant problems can develop in the relationship of an IMG physician and female nurses or co-workers. It is not uncommon to hear sexist remarks from some IMGs. Some may even consider American women loose because of their seemingly provocative dress.

As a resident one day while I was making hospital rounds, I overhead a group of nurses talking. The discussion was about several of the resident doctors on unit, all of which were IMGs. One very disgusted nurse asked, 'Why does he always look at me like I'm a piece of meat?' It took a while before I realized the dynamics of what was going on and what was meant by that question. Because of the friendly outgoing nature of American women, coupled with the different style of clothing, these new IMGs were misinterpreting the intentions of these nurses.

It is to the benefit of the IMG physician to learn about and understand these cultural variables as soon as possible. I would urge all IMGs to read about male/female relationships in the workplace and become familiar with the term 'sexual harassment' before you find yourself in more trouble than you ever imagined.

MEDICAL EDUCATION

'Life is short, and the act long, occasion instant, experiment perilous, decision difficult' (Hippocrates).

Love of learning is the philosophy on which medicine is based[10]. A physician must have the drive and will to learn. With such a resolve, graduates (the residents) will practice medicine competently; without it, no amount of acquired information will help. Physicians must express their desire in hard and continuing work, as well as frequently working hard when they do not feel like it; consider this course to be a training exercise of the will. For the effective practice of medicine, teamwork, honesty, kindness, awareness and concern for others are all clearly essential.

Each medical encounter will remain unique. The physician will still struggle to bring the wisdom of the ages to an individual person in a complex, ambiguous and always new situation, even when there is advanced technology around us. Learning will continue to be the basis of medicine[10,11].

Experience, training, qualification and continuing education are all related to the more technical aspects of medical practice. While it is true that all of these factors play a role in self-development, one of the most significant and often most overlooked factors is interpersonal skills[12]. Simply put, interpersonal skills determine how we get along with people. All significant appointments and opinions of our peers, as well as our patients, are influenced by interpersonal skills. Our medical schools and residency training programs are filled with high achievers, and yet this is the very group that has little time for social activity and hence they often lack these important skills[13]. I am often told by my residents, 'It's not in my personality to hold my patient's hand.' My response to that is, 'If you were not born with this skill, then you better develop it.'

PATIENT–PHYSICIAN RELATIONSHIPS

Patient dissatisfaction is at an all time high. In a recent public opinion poll conducted by the American Medical Association, only 60% of the patients surveyed were very satisfied with their own physician[14]. An even smaller percentage was satisfied with the medical profession in general. One way to reverse this alarming trend of increasing patient dissatisfaction, is to train our young physicians in the development of interpersonal skills. These skills include the art of listening, attentiveness, temper and emotion control, voice control and body language, as well as becoming familiar with and more tolerant of people from various backgrounds, cultures, educational levels and temperament. Always remember that physicians are in the business of making people feel better. Developing these skills will go a long way in achieving that result. Some of the more common reasons given for patient dissatisfaction are that physicians spend too little time with their patients and that they do not explain things very well. Patients often perceive (and rightfully so) that physicians are in a hurry to get out of the examining room and are really more interested in making money than in the care of their patients[11,12].

Patients' emotional needs

It is important that the biomedical as well as the emotional needs of the patient are met in order for the patient to be truly satisfied. Martin and Bass[15] found that patients who believed that 'the doctor tells me all I want to know about my illness,' and 'the doctor gives me a chance to say what is really on my mind,' felt that they were helped, were more satisfied, and had a higher rate of compliance. Furthermore, the patient's evaluation of the physician's affective tone or ability to discuss psychological issues probably affects the evaluation of the physician's biomedical abilities[12].

Improving the relationship

Simple steps can be taken to make patients feel that you have time for them and that you care about them. Try sitting down — even for a minute! Sit on a stool next to them, or on the side of the bed — somewhere close to the patient. Try touching your patients. Look them straight in the eye while talking and listening to them. Give them your full attention. Do not keep looking at the chart or keep a hand on the door knob! These are all simple but extremely helpful ways to make your patient feel that he or she is the most important thing on your mind. Before leaving the examination room, ask the patient, 'Can I answer any other questions for you?', or, 'Can I do something else today to make you more comfortable?' These simple acts can go a long way in alleviating the perception of too little time and too little caring. A colleague of mine mastered this art and consequently was loved and revered by his patients. While visiting a patient, he would always sit down on the bedside, touch the patient with his hand, and then take out an old pipe and pretend to be cleaning it. This made him seem a little more human and endeared him a bit more to his patients.

Another factor that contributes to a poor physician–patient relationship is the excessive use of medical terminology. Patients may not understand the terminology, so a physician should use plain and simple English. Furthermore, important facts and information should be repeated several times, then ask the patient to repeat back what you have told him to be sure that he understands what you are trying to say. A physician must practice these techniques for developing a better relationship with his patients. A physician who cannot communicate well with his patients is working in a vacuum. Ineffective communication can be confusing and frustrating for the patient. The positive end-result of good communication is very rewarding for the physician as well as the patient[16,17]. In the complex liability atmosphere of today it is becoming more and more apparent that a patient who is well-satisfied with his physician is less apt to file a malpractice suit against that physician[18].

PATHWAY TO SUCCESS

We have discussed the general aspects of self-development and the importance of a good patient–physician relationship. I would now like to share with you some of my thoughts on enhancing self-development and improving the patient–physician relationship. This, in turn, will hopefully provide you with some direction so that you can discover your own meaning of success.

It is quite easy and comfortable for any physician to stay in his narrow circle of acquaintances and friends, but to be successful one has to widen one's horizons.

I had to make a conscious decision to widen my horizons and learn to participate in activities outside the practice of medicine. It was quite easy once I made the decision to participate in the affairs of organized medicine. It was immediately apparent to me that there were a lot of people ready to help and I was received with open arms.

I read, listened and actively participated. I knew that if I wanted to play a role in my destiny, that is, to promote the practice of medicine and its future, I must participate.

It was not long after that day, that my colleagues at the Wayne County Medical Society (Detroit, Michigan) were nominating me to run for the position of president of the fourth largest county medical society in the US. In 1989 I became the first IMG president of this distinguished organization with a membership of more than 4000. It was truly a great honor.

Since then I have had the pleasure of holding multiple significant positions, both at the County and State Society in Michigan and the American Medical Association.

In 1993 I felt greatly honored when the International College of Surgeons US Section, an organization with approximately 16 000 surgeon members, elected me as their Regent of the Year. The same year I was also elected as the Founding President of the Michigan Chapter. For the last 15 years I have served as the Chief of Surgery and the Director of Medical Education at a 300-bed community hospital.

The reason to share a few things about myself is not to tell you how great I am, but to emphasize that we can achieve anything in the US if we want to. Being an IMG should not hold you down and it should not be used as an excuse. One should try hard to rise above 'just being an IMG' to becoming a successful American physician.

The list of accomplishments by IMG physicians is long. Until recently, both the Chairmen of the Departments of Surgery and Medicine at Wayne State University in Detroit were IMGs. Throughout the US, many department chairmen are IMGs. With a lot of hard work and then overcoming various obstacles, you *can* become a successful physician in the US. Some of the following points which I have learned and found beneficial I would like to share with you.

Develop your ability to listen

Research has shown that on the average, physicians only give 12 seconds to a patient before they start speaking or asking questions[11]. It is no wonder that patients complain that physicians do not listen to them. The failure to listen to our patients is not only rude and disrespectful, it can actually lead to misdiagnosis.

The art of 'good listening' can also have positive effects outside of the workplace. People who really listen when another person is talking are held in higher esteem.

There are no hidden secrets to becoming a great listener. Give the speaker your complete undivided attention and look him in the eye when he is talking. Allow him to fully and completely explain his condition and ask if he has any questions. The ability to listen is a learned behavior and requires a conscious effort and diligent practice. When you start learning new things from others, and realize you know a lot less than you once thought you did, you probably are on your way to becoming a good listener.

Determination and persistence

Most celebrities and millionaires have one thing in common; they tried and failed numerous times before they reached their goals and found success. Do not be afraid to fail, for through our failures can we find success. Calvin Coolidge once said:

> 'Nothing in the world can take the place of persistence. Talent will not. Nothing is more common than unsuccessful men with great talent. Genius will not, unrewarded genius is almost intolerable. Education will not. The world is full of educated derelicts. Persistence and determination alone are omnipotent.'

Maintain a sense of humor

Humor is good medicine. A good laugh releases tension and can get those endorphines circulating. Physicians are finally agreeing with this idea. In fact, some medical organizations around the nation are now committed to bringing more humor into medicine. We all know that medicine is a tough business and can generate high levels of stress.

A successful physician will learn to get out of tough situations by using a little humor. Learn to laugh at yourself. People enjoy being around humorous people. We all know how infectious laughter can be. The 'joke teller' always has an audience. Do not take life so seriously that you cannot enjoy all of the beauty and happiness around you.

Learn to dress well/personal hygiene

John T. Molloy has done extensive research on how to dress for success[19]. His research has shown that in the hospital setting, the physician's white coat is viewed as a symbol of power. He also demonstrated, however, that that symbol of power disappears once the physician moves outside of those hospital walls.

Physicians are often not considered to be good dressers. Mr Molloy feels strongly that all professionals, including physicians, should dress well. For men, dark suits with ties emit success. Shoes must be clean and polished. Women face special problems, according to Mr Molloy. They should wear dark suits with skirts below the knee in length. Non-Western apparel will usually shift attention to the clothes and away from the topic of discussion. Recent immigrants to the US often encounter this problem. Every attempt should be made to switch to Western style dress as soon as possible, at least in professional situations. If you dress like a foreigner, you will be treated like one. Non-Western dress may not hurt you, but will rarely help you.

Whether or not you embrace the rules of John T. Molloy, I think a few simple ideas should be remembered. Being well dressed does not mean that your clothes are flashy, expensive and custom-made. Clean, well laundered, and properly fitting clothes are best. One does not have to wear the latest fashion trend to be well dressed, but I would discourage wearing 'bell bottoms' to an interview. It is my experience that successful people usually dress well. This is one of the simplest ways, at least initially, to get the interest, attention and respect of others. First impressions do make a difference.

I think it is also important to stress a point on personal hygiene. It may seem so basic as to be silly. In America, millions of dollars are spent every year on personal hygiene products. There is a special dislike for the smell of sweat and other body odors. Deodorants, antiperspirants, colognes, mouthwash and breath fresheners are all important and are an integral part of American personal hygiene.

Everybody is expected to take a shower daily, use deodorant and antiperspirant under each arm before getting dressed with a clean shirt, and brush their teeth twice daily to avoid bad breath and tooth problems. The use of after-shave lotions and colognes can also be very helpful.

I have never forgotten the day my chief told me I had body odor. It came to me as a surprise, as I considered myself very clean and well-dressed. The problem was I had never learned to use deodorants and antiperspirants. I learned this lesson fast and not a day probably goes by when I do not think of it and thank my chief; he may have changed my life. Every day we encounter people who have offensive body odor. If you know someone who has this problem, one of the kindest and most helpful things you can do for that person is discretely and gently tell them about it. Chances are, he will be forever grateful to you.

Enthusiasm

Be enthusiastic about life. I look forward to each new day (granted, I look forward to some more than others). Whenever I find myself getting tired and discouraged, I try to see the world through the eyes of my baby daughter. When she wakes up in the morning, sleep barely wiped from her eyes, she leaps up in her crib to stare outside the window. The rustling leaves, the soaring birds and the playful squirrels hold such a fascination for her. She can hardly wait to start her day, anticipating the wonders she will discover in the new day's adventures. Norman Vincent Peale described enthusiasm the best.

> 'Enthusiasm develops and maintains the quality of determination which helps you overcome fear and builds self-confidence, and enthusiasm can induce the powerful motivation that makes things happen. Enthusiasm makes the difference between success and failure. Enthusiasm is contagious and it makes other people enthusiastic. Anything done with enthusiasm has a better chance of being accomplished. People who do things with enthusiasm suddenly are placed in a higher category than others.[20]'

Overcome feelings of inferiority

Zig Zigler, author of multiple best-seller 'self-help' books, has written extensively about the inferiority complex. He states that approximately 95% of all people experience feelings of inferiority at some time in their life. These feelings can be related to education, personal appearance and money. Some people cannot even explain why they feel inferior[21].

Residency training is a competitive learning situation where you are frequently called upon to demonstrate your knowledge and competency before peers and supervisors. Hence, the learning situation itself becomes one of the most intense anxiety-provoking situations of life[3]. Feelings of inferiority probably came to the surface on a daily, sometimes hourly, basis. This myriad of emotions and feelings leads to a depletion of energy which produces more stress and even deeper feelings of inferiority. It can be a vicious downward spiraling cycle. If feelings of inferiority start to interfere with your ability to function effectively, try to identify the source of the feelings. Then focus on all of your positive traits and characteristics. Pat yourself on the back when you accomplish something. If you make a conscious effort to do this every day, feelings of inferiority will soon be replaced with feelings of security[21].

A gratifying professional life, a satisfying social life and a happy family life are important. It is imperative that you find time for your spouse and children. The amount of time and attention that you give will be rewarded many times over. Do take time off from work. Vacations for pleasure are not a waste of time.

Explore the theaters, symphony, art museums and other activities such as PTA (Parent Teacher Association) groups and church activities. It is important to get involved in other activities beyond the practice of medicine. If you are afraid to wander too far outside the medical realm, get involved in organized medicine. At least you will get away from your everyday duties and responsibilities and you probably will learn something new in the process. Who knows? You might even enjoy it!

CONCLUSIONS

To be a good and successful physician is like climbing Mount Everest. It can be done, but needs training and patience. You need to be knowledgeable, hard working, patient, receptive, a moderator, secure, a careful planner, a good listener, a leader and sympathetic to patients. Physicians are expected to be kind, courteous, and have honesty and integrity. For them, the welfare of the patient always comes first. Men and women have already achieved this, as is evident from the scores of good and successful physicians all around us. Younger physicians should carefully observe and learn from these 'role models'.

One definition of success which I have always cherished was written by Bessie Anderson Stanley in 1904.

'He has achieved success who has lived well, laughed often and loved much; who has enjoyed the trust of pure woman, the respect of intelligent men and the love of little children; who has filled his niche and accomplished his task; who has left the world better than he found it, whether an improved poppy, perfect poem or a rescued soul; who has always looked for the best in others and given them the best he had; whose life was an inspiration; whose memory a benediction.'[22]

REFERENCES

1. Robock, A., Randolph, L. and Seidman, B. (1992). *Physician Characteristics Distribution in the US.* (Chicago: American Medical Association)
2. Havelwala, Y. A. (1979). Problems of foreign born psychiatrists. *Psychiatr. Q.*, **51**, 307–12
3. Gavinia, M. and Wintrob, R. (1975). Foreign medical graduates who return home after US residency training — the Peruvian case. *J. Med. Educ.*, **50**, 167–75

4. Committee on Ways and Means. (1986). *The Hidden Agenda: New York State Retrictions on Foreign Medical Schools.* (New York: New York Assembly)
5. Shuval, J. T. (1985). Social functions of medical licensing: a case study of Soviet immigrant physicians in Israel. *Soc. Sci. Med.,* **20,** 901–9
6. Rhee, S. O., Lyons, T. F., Payne, B. C. and Moskowitz, S. E. (1986). USMG's and FMG's: are there performance differences in the ambulatory care setting? *Med. Care,* **24,** 248–58
7. Holberstam, J. L., Antler, L., Rush H. A. and Seltzer, J. D. (1971). Foreign interns in community hospitals. *J. Med. Educ.,* **46,** 504
8. Norcini, J. J., Shea, J. A. and Benson, J. A. (1991). Changes in the medical knowledge of candidates for certification. *Ann. Intern. Med.,* **114,** 33–5
9. Rosner, F. and Mulvihill, J. E. (1979). American foreign medical graduates performance after a year of supervised clinical clerkship (fifth pathway). *J. Am. Med. Assoc.,* **241,** 714–16
10. Tosteson, D. C. (1979). Learning in medicine. *N. Engl. J. Med.,* **301,** 690–4
11. Bertakis, K. D., Roter, D. and Putnam, S. M. (1991). The relationship of physician medical interview style to patient satisfaction. *J. Fam. Pract.,* **32,** 175–81
12. Bowman, M. A. (1991). Good physician–patient relationship = improved patient outcome. *J. Fam. Pract.,* **32,** 135–6
13. Huxham, G. J., Lipton, A. and Hamilton, D. (1989). What 'makes' a good doctor? *Med. Educ.,* **23,** 3–13
14. American Medical Association. (1991). *Public Opinion on Health Care Issues 1991.* (Chicago, IL: Department of Issues and Communication Research)
15. Martin, F. J. and Bass, M. J. (1989). The impact of discussion of nonmedical problems in the physician's office. *Fam. Pract.,* **6,** 254–8
16. Arnold, R. M. and Forrow, L. (1990). Rewarding medicine: good doctors and good behavior. *Ann. Intern. Med.,* **113,** 794–8
17. Witmer, J. M. (1985). *Pathways to Personal Growth.* (Muncie, IN: Accelerated Development Inc.)
18. Kusserow, R. P., Handley, E. A. and Yessian, M. R. (1987). An overview of state medical discipline. *J. Am. Med. Assoc.,* **257,** 820–4
19. Molloy, J. T. (1988). *New Dress For Success.* (New York: Warner Books)
20. Peale, N. V. (1967). *Enthusiasm Makes the Difference.* (Englewood, NJ: Prentice Hall Inc.)
21. Zigler, Z. (1990). *Steps to the Top.* (Gretna: Pelican Publishing Company)
22. Stanley, B. A. (1904). Quote. In *Ann Lander's Column, Detroit Free Press, June 1991,* B2

11

Medical education: a lifelong process

R. J. Kiel and S. A. Phillips

INTRODUCTION

Your medical education does not stop after medical school and residency. What ends abruptly is the passive learner's method of acquiring knowledge; what must begin is the active acquisition of information by a learner who is self-motivated to seek knowledge on his own. The following chapter is divided into two parts. The first section is devoted to a discussion regarding the best ways to learn, followed by a second section which discusses the optimal use of the medical library.

AN EFFECTIVE METHOD OF LIFELONG ADULT LEARNING

The best physicians are self-directed, life-long learners. They realize early in their careers that the traditional lecture-based format of continuing medical education (CME) is an ineffective method of self-directed adult learning. Outstanding physicians develop methods of learning and do it efficiently. The following chapter will give you some tips on how adults learn efficiently after leaving school.

Physicians progress through several phases of educational development. Knowles[1] has proposed a theory of adult education, which is summarized in Table 11-1. Initially, learning occurs through interaction between an expert instructor and a fact-deficient student: the pedagogical model of learning. This flow of information is one way, dictated by the instructor. The format begins in grade school and persists through the first 2 years of medical school.

Table 11-1. Models of learning

Traditional learning — the pedagogical model:
Learner is dependent; teacher decides what is to be learned
Learners have little experience on which to build new knowledge
Learning is a sequential process of acquiring new subject matter
Motivation to learn is external through parents and teachers, etc.

Adult learning — the andragogical model:
The learner is self directed; he is *responsible* for his education
Adults bring past experiences to the learning encounter; adults learn best
    from each other
Learning is problem-centered or task-centered in orientation
Adults are motivated to learn by internal forces: self-esteem, greater
    self-confidence and recognition

Testing is fact-based and encourages rote memorization and retrieval upon command. Incentives for learning include getting a passing grade on examinations and promotion to higher academic levels.

In adult education, learning goals are different than in the traditional learning model. Learning is centered around solution of problems; motivation for learning is internal. The responsibility for learning is centered on the individual.

Once you leave the structured environment of medical school, learning goals, by necessity, change. Professional needs include providing the best care for patients and keeping your knowledge base updated. One can satisfy these learning objectives through attendance at traditional CME courses, through interaction with colleagues, by reading medical journals and textbooks, or through other activities of dependent learning (audio or video cassettes, computer interactive instruction and small group discussions, etc.).

Audio tapes are an excellent alternative to the lecture-based format. Many speakers are taped at national meetings discussing the most current topics. The educational material is usually distilled to its essence because of constraints of the speaker's allowed time. Some physicians do the bulk of their continuing education by listening to tapes in their cars on the way to work.

The traditional lecture-based CME course (or the audio cassettes of it) does not provide the most effective medium to satisfy the broad goals of physician education. Fact-based lectures are not interactive, do not result in any change in health care outcomes of patients[2] and do not promote long-term retention of facts or concepts. Physicians, in our experience, learn best when they are motivated to do it. They need to learn to structure, integrate and apply new knowledge using a patient-based domain. Physicians must be self-directed, lifelong learners.

Educational reform in medical schools

In the 1980s, recommendations were made by national advisory committees concerning the improvement of the professional education of physicians. Several of the key recommendations with reference to medical schools were recently reviewed in a report by Swanson and Anderson[3]. A major focus was to develop active, independent, self-directed learning skills in medical students and to decrease the use of lectures. Students were encouraged to learn independently in order to prepare themselves for a lifetime of continued growth and development. If medical students are encouraged to be independent learners, postgraduate CME programs must continue that emphasis and provide opportunities for active, self-directed learning. The best way to accomplish this goal is to read about the symptoms and diseases of your patients.

Adult learning

Adults learn through the acquisition, encoding and elaboration of knowledge[4,5]. *Acquisition* involves integrating new material into a structural framework formed by past knowledge of the subject. Learning techniques should be designed to review and update the knowledge base of the participant before new information is presented. The process of *encoding* involves learning a subject in a similar environment in which recall will be needed. As an example, physicians should read about the diseases present in the patients at the nursing station rather than in the library the next day. Clinical rounds and teaching should be done at the patient's bedside as this is the environment where the information will be used in the future. Once information is acquired and encoded, *elaboration* of the information in the form of discussion, question and answer sessions or teaching by peers yields a greater understanding of the subject material.

Fact-based lectures: optimal utilization. Each physician should first determine what educational techniques work best for him. The traditional, fact-based lecture is most familiar. This method of education tends to be one-sided; participants are for the most part passive listeners. This forum may be good for presentation of novel research techniques or new information, but as a vehicle of learning for the physician, lectures do not result in long-term retention of concepts or change patient outcomes[2].

To best utilize the traditional lecture-based CME format, the physician must be actively involved. Education activities should be chosen that are both interesting and relevant to his or her practice of medicine. The physician should commit some time to reading about the subject prior to the lecture; he should take notes during the lecture, ask pertinent questions following the presentation, and attempt to integrate the subject material into his personal knowledge base. Finally, he should assess his understanding of the subject material by self-assessment techniques such as recertification examinations. This process takes considerable effort and, we believe, is not one that most physicians would be motivated to continue.

Problem-based learning. An alternative to the traditional CME activity is problem-based learning (PBL), which employs patient scenarios to stimulate discussion about the diagnostic approach to a clinical situation[6]. Participants discuss the pathophysiology involved in the disease process under the guidance of a facilitator. Finally, the best approach to solving the problem is developed.

The problem-based educational technique is interactive and stimulates the acquisition of new knowledge. By forming a framework for new information, it is more fully retained and, through interactions between participants, physicians can practice using this new information. The basic principles of adult education (acquisition, encoding and elaboration of knowledge) are satisfied.

Physicians as adult learners

That a physician's knowledge base deteriorates over time[7] should come as no surprise. There is a significant inverse correlation between examination scores and the number of years since certification in medicine. Traditional CME activities do not correlate with performance on examinations, unlike the reading of medical journals[7]. Perhaps this educational activity best reflects the dedication of the individual physician to actively expand his or her knowledge base and the desire for self-directed learning.

A survey of physicians' views on the contribution of different education phases to practice performance[8] uncovered striking results. Most participants felt that specialty education and practice-based independent learning were superior to university education and traditional CME methods in their daily practice. Twenty-three per cent of physicians felt that formal CME made no contribution to their knowledge or skills. All physicians with board certification whose licenses were issued in 1985 or earlier, stated that they participated in self-organized study groups. Traditional fact-based lectures (both in medical school and in traditional CME) were felt to contribute the least to the practicing physicians' knowledge base. These studies suggest that physicians need to update their knowledge base as new information arises. Self-directed study may be the best way to accomplish this goal.

Clinical reasoning: how clinicians become experts
The development of a physician's knowledge base occurs in stages.

Principle based. Initially, medical knowledge is fact based and consists of physiological and pathophysiological principles that are separate and unlinked. Subsequently, facts become linked through a cause and effect relationship. A student responding to the problem of a patient with chest pain would draw upon his knowledge of the pathophysiology of myocardial ischemia and dermatomal representation of visceral pain.

Disease-presentation based. Once patients are interviewed, the student doctor must relate the patient's varied symptom complex to known pathophysiological processes. His or her knowledge base reorganizes and evaluates on the basis of disease presentations. Symptoms are explained on the basis of physiological processes and new knowledge is associated with predefined models of disease. These models of disease provide a framework on to which new seemingly diverse facts can be hung and remembered. Once the physician has seen several patients with a particular disease, he constructs his own 'illness scripts'[9] which characterize the varied presentation of patients with a particular disease.

Each illness script consists of enabling conditions (predisposing factors, demographic data and hereditary data), the malfunction that allows disease to occur (invasion of tissue by a microorganism and ischemia of tissue) and the consequences of the illness (signs, symptoms and abnormal laboratory data).

Knowledge structure becomes centered on the symptoms and signs of disease rather than on fact-based or causal theory. Subsequent problem solving entails matching a patient's presentation with the previously constructed scripts of disease. Further data acquisition either confirms or refutes the illness in question. As clinicians have contact with more patients, elaborate scripts are constructed and clinical reasoning is enriched.

Patient-experience based. After a physician has been professionally involved with many patients, he begins to structure his knowledge around memories of individual patients. For example: a model of systemic lupus erythematosus (SLE) emerges from a compilation of two or three patients. New information about SLE is linked to this patient representation. Recall of information about lupus will elicit a vivid recall of individual patients. The more patients the physician cares for, the more elaborate the cognitive scaffold. Learning is related to the clinical situation: a patient with SLE will invoke knowledge learned at the bedside of the last patient with SLE.

Clinical-based learning: the clinical paradigm

Physicians may need to learn about new diseases without the benefit of patient contact. Rare diseases like dermatomyositis or α_1-antitrypsin deficiency are important for the young clinician to recognize, yet often are not represented in their patient mix. A concept that I have found useful is to construct a clinical paradigm that summarizes the usual presentation of

---

Clinical paradigm for dermatomyositis

This is a middle aged woman who presents with the insidious onset of proximal muscle weakness and an aching pain in the muscles. There was no double vision. The patient complained of a lilac-colored heliotrope rash on the eyelids. There was a facial rash on the bridge of the nose in a butterfly distribution. A scaling dermatitis was present on the knuckles. The patient complained of mild dysphagia and was diagnosed by a cardiologist to have a resolving myocarditis.

Upon physical examination, there was periorbital edema. Weakness of the proximal muscles was noted but there was no change in the reflexes. A rash with ulceration was noticed on the fingers near the nail beds.

On laboratory examination, CPK and aldolase were elevated, as was SGOT or LDH. ANA was positive and myoglobin was seen in the urine. Skeletal muscle biopsy showed infiltration of inflammatory cells with destruction of muscle fibers. Anti-Jo-1 antibody was negative.

Figure 11-1. An example of a clinical paradigm.
CPK, creatine phosphokinase; SGOT, serum glutamic oxalo-acetic transaminase; LDH, lactate dehydrogenase; ANA, antinuclear antibody

a patient in a narrative format. This clinical paradigm allows the young clinician to construct a 'cognitive patient' that can be utilized to structure future knowledge of the disease. Rereading prior clinical paradigms should yield greater retention of the disease process than the review of a set of facts on the disease that are not yet woven together. An example of a clinical paradigm is presented in Figure 11-1.

Conclusions

Physicians in practice learn differently than as students and residents. They graduate from a passive, pedagogical lecture format of learning to a self-directed interactive lifetime learner. As a physician you have a responsibility constantly to update your knowledge base. This chapter has provided some tips on how to make this transition. A synopsis of effective learning techniques is summarized below.

How to learn efficiently
(1) Have a firm commitment to improve your medical knowledge every day. Doctors who want to learn will do it well.

(2) Assess what learning technique you prefer best: lecture-based format, computer interactive instruction, small group discussions, PBL, or independent reading of journals or textbooks.

(3) Prepare for a lecture-based presentation by reading about the subject matter; take notes during the lecture and attempt to use the new information by asking questions of the presenter.

(4) Remain inquisitive; challenge past dictums with an open mind.

(5) Become an effective teacher of medical students, interns, residents or fellow staff members. Try to use an interactive format with your group. 'To teach is to learn twice.'[10]

(6) Read and investigate the medical literature as it applies to your patients.

(7) Volunteer to take recertification examinations.

(8) Attempt to organize new information into a patient-based clinical paradigm (Figure 11-1) which consists of a patient profile that integrates the major presenting features, the exacerbating conditions and the main

diagnostic features of an illness. By constructing and rereading this paradigm, factual information will be integrated and retained.

THE MEDICAL LIBRARY AND SELF-DIRECTED LEARNING

The previous section discussed the limitations of lecture format CME as the model for physician postgraduate education. Weinberg and colleagues have noted that physicians have rated highly the educational benefits accrued through learning from colleagues and self-directed learning via journals. Much of the self-directed learning necessary as a practicing physician may be found at your hospital medical library.

The sheer volume of the medical literature has made traditional information seeking methods such as browsing through office collections of printed books and journal subscriptions too inefficient to be effective[12,13]. Electronic information retrieval services available through most hospital libraries can help streamline your information access needs. These services include Medline and database searching, delivery of journal articles from in-house collections, and interlibrary loan, in which journal articles and books are obtained from other libraries. Some hospital libraries offer alerting services, such as journal routing and table of contents services. Updating services such as Selective Dissemination of Information (SDI) are also available.

If your local hospital does not provide library services, you should contact the nearest medical school or large hospital library. Frequently these libraries provide the aforementioned services on a fee for service basis either by telephone, US mail, telefacsimile or electronic mail.

Accessing hospital library services

An essential question to be asked about the hospital library is whether and how it can be accessed from remote locations such as the office or home. Many hospital libraries, and most medical school libraries, have electronic catalogs containing their book and journal collections. In many cases, these catalogs can be accessed from a physician's home or office through the hospital's electronic network, or by using a computer, modem and special dial-in software. Increasingly, requests for Medline searches, books and journal articles can be requested in this way. Regardless of the size of the hospital's library collection, electronic networks and telefacsimile technology have made it possible for the resources of libraries across the country to be delivered directly to the physician's office, often within hours of the request.

Textbooks and CD/ROM

Textbooks and similar types of reference materials are useful sources of background, factual or drug information. They are useful for finding overview or background discussions of medical conditions and diagnostic/treatment methodologies. While these types of books continue as a mainstay of the medical library, increasingly, they are found in electronic format, in the form of CD/ROM (compact disk, read-only-memory). A form of optical disk technology, CD/ROM offers many benefits over printed texts. It allows much more information to be stored in a compact fashion, permits the entire text to be searched by keyword, and may be accessed through remote computers and shared among several users at the same time. For office use, physicians may find that CD/ROM formats offer all these advantages. However, CD/ROM texts pose a problem for users as the electronic formats require a software program to access the text, and because different CD/ROM vendors use different software which may leave first-time users feeling confused or frustrated. Library staff generally are familiar with the various CD/ROM software packages, and can be helpful in explaining how a program works, or in assisting you with other types of problems. If you are considering purchasing CD/ROM resources for your home or office, consider previewing the product, either through a demonstration arrangement with the vendor, or seeing the product in operation in the library or in a colleague's office, etc. The CD/ROM medical products are demonstrated frequently at medical meetings where exhibit areas are featured. It is also important to have examined any documentation or user manuals, etc., which accompany the product, in order to determine which hardware best serves your needs.

Journal literature

Journal literature is the medium through which scientists and physicians first report new medical and scientific information. The importance of regularly consulting the journal literature in the usual course of patient care is discussed by several authors[14-16], although the same authors agree that the sheer volume of the literature requires a well-constructed strategy. Haynes *et al.*[17] suggest identifying the core journals which can be scanned regularly. They also suggest that you get to know the hospital librarian. Through their knowledge of the journal literature and electronic retrieval systems, librarians can help analyze your information needs and set up systems for identifying relevant articles.

Medline

The primary electronic means of accessing the medical journal literature is through use of Medline. Medline, the National Library of Medicine's (NLMs) major bibliographic database, contains more than 900 000 citations to the recent medical journal literature and indexes over 3000 biomedical and health-related journals. Updated weekly, Medline can provide searches of material which was published as far back as 1966.

The benefits of Medline vary with the nature of the information needed. Clinicians consult Medline to support clinical patient care decisions; they also may search the literature to compile a bibliography for a research or publication project. Whatever the purpose of the search, the requester receives a list of articles on the subject, including abstracts if they are requested.

Medline is actually one of several biomedical databases available through NLM's MEDLARS (Medical Literature Analysis and Retrieval System). These databases include information on toxicology, health planning and administration, cancer research and several other areas. Your librarian can provide a complete list of these databases and recommend those appropriate for your needs.

In most hospitals, Medline is a major service offered by the medical library. You can request a Medline search to be performed by a trained medical librarian, or you can perform your own Medline search through use of one of several available end-user Medline systems.

Searching Medline as an end-user. End-user or requester Medline systems are do-it-yourself Medline programs designed to lead you, the requester, through a search session using a desktop computer and special search software. Most hospital libraries provide end-user Medline search services through a computer in the library itself; in many libraries, it also is possible to perform an end-user Medline search from your office or home through a computer and modem.

Success in performing a Medline search as an end-user lies in becoming familiar with the system's software, and in developing an understanding of how the Medline database is organized. Numerous end-user systems exist, and each one has its own organization and command system. Albright[18] and Siegel *et al.*[19] provide useful introductions to on-line bibliographic searching for physicians. Medical libraries frequently provide end-user training sessions, search manuals, and other types of searching tools which can make the search process easier. Medical librarians are familiar with most end-user Medline systems and

Table 11-2. Medline vendors

BRS Colleague, BRS Information Technologies, 800 West Park Drive, McLean, Virginia 22102, USA. (Tel: 800-955-0406.)	Grateful Med, National Technical Information Services, 5285 Port Royal Road, Springfield, Virginia 22161, USA. (Tel: 800-638-8480.)
CD-Plus, CD-Plus Technologies, 333 Seventh Avenue, 6th Floor, New York, New York 10001, USA. (Tel: 800-950-2035.)	PaperChase, Longwood Galleria, 350 Longwood Avenue, Boston, Massachusetts 02115, USA. (Tel: 800-722-2075.)
Compact Cambridge Medline, Cambridge Scientific Abstracts, 7200 Wisconsin Avenue, Bethesda, Maryland 20814, USA. (Tel: 301-961-6700.)	SilverPlatter Medline, SilverPlatter Information Inc., 37 Walnut Street, Wellesley Hills, Massachusetts 02181, USA. (Tel: 617-239-0306.)

can help trouble-shoot search strategy problems and search mechanics. A selective list of end-user systems is: BRS Colleague, CD-Plus, Compact Cambridge Medline, Grateful Med, PaperChase and SilverPlatter Medline. Their addresses are listed in Table 11-2.

Obtaining/managing journal articles. A Medline search produces a printed list of references to journal articles. Depending on the Medline system used, the printout may include abstracts. In any case, there arrives a point at which the physician wants to read an article which is not available in his or her own office collection. These articles can be obtained conveniently and quickly by contacting your hospital library. Most libraries can provide articles for physicians either from in-house journal collections, or through interlibrary loan.

Through electronic access and telefacsimile technology, requested articles can be in the physician's hands within the same day of request. The advantage of obtaining articles through the hospital library is that the service is generally provided free of charge. If your hospital does not provide library services, you may try contacting the nearest medical school library or large hospital library. Frequently, these libraries will provide you with articles on a fee for service basis. Articles can also be obtained through various commercial arrangements, but you are charged several dollars for each article. Some end-user Medline systems, such as BRS Colleague and Grateful Med (see Table 11-2), provide a means of ordering articles on-line at the end of your search. These services also charge substantial fees for delivery of articles, but can be useful if your hospital does not provide article delivery services through the library.

Current awareness and alerting services

Several current awareness services designed to assist physicians in keeping up to date with the newly published journal literature also exist. *Current Contents* is an excellent subscription service which provides contents pages from a broad range of biomedical journal titles. Haynes et al.[20] also suggest selective dissemination of information (SDI) services for physicians with highly specialized interests, as these provide a means whereby a specific subject profile is stored in the Medline computer. The physician then receives a monthly printed bibliography on a highly relevant topic. The SDI service is available from the hospital library, or from commercial vendors such as Dialog and BRS. Commercial vendors charge fees for these services. Your hospital's medical library can explain which types of these services may best suit your needs.

Computer-assisted instruction

Computer-Assisted Instruction (CAI) uses computer technology to provide interactive programmed learning experiences on focused topics or skills. The CAI programs typically take the form of case simulations in which the physician is presented with a set of symptoms or conditions, and is asked to choose from among a list of diagnostic and/or treatment methodologies. The program responds to the choices made by the user, providing interactive feedback on the student's answers. Incorrect answers are provided with additional screens to help correct the choice; correct answers permit the user to go on with the program, or ask for additional information. Computer-Assisted Instruction programs are available on a broad range of subjects, and as with CD/ROM products, they tend to vary as to their ease of use and presentation format. Usually, CAI programs are accompanied by user manuals, which tend to be of variable quality.

Some CAI products are produced on floppy disk, while others utilize CD/ROM technology. Recent developments in CAI involve the use of interactive videodisk technology to integrate images with computer-based teaching programs. Use of interactive videodisks, or multimedia, permit combined use of a variety of media such as X-ray and radiographic images, histology slides, videotaped patient sessions and explanatory text, etc. Hoffer and Barnett[21] provide additional information on current and future trends in computer-assisted instruction.

SUMMARY

One thing is certain in your career; medical information will change. Continuing medical education will be among the most important activities in your medical practice. Your challenge as an adult learner will be to transform from the passive medical student into an active, self-directed learner. Use of the information resources and services presented in this chapter can help you achieve this goal.

REFERENCES

1. Knowles, M. S. (1984). *Androgogy in Action: Applying Modern Principles of Adult Learning.* (San Francisco: Jossey-Bass Publishers)
2. Davis, D. A., Thomson, M. A., Oxman, A. D. and Haynes, R. B. (1992). Evidence for the effectiveness of CME: a review of 50 randomized controlled trials. *J. Am. Med. Assoc.,* **268,** 1111–17
3. Swanson, A. G. and Anderson M. B. (1993). Educating medical students: assessing change in medical education — the road to implementation. *Acad. Med.,* **68,** S1–65
4. Schmidt, H. G. (1983). Problem based learning: rationale and description. *Med. Educ.,* **17,** 11–16
5. Albanese, M. A. and Mitchell, S. (1993). Problem-based learning: a review of literature on its outcomes and implementation issues. *Acad. Med.,* **68,** 52-81
6. Norman, G. R. and Schmidt, H. G. (1992). The psychological basis of problem-based learning: a review of the evidence. *Acad. Med.,* **67,** 557–65
7. Ramsey, P. G., Carline, J. D., Inui, T. S., Larsau, E. B., Logerfo, J. P., Norcini, J. J. and Wenrich, M. D. (1991). Changes over time in the knowledge base of practicing internists. *J. Am. Med. Assoc.,* **266,** 1103–7

8. Renschler, H. E. and Fuchs, U. (1993). Lifelong learning of physicians: contributions of different educational phases to practice performance. *Acad. Med.,* **68,** S57–9

9. Schmidt, H. G., Norman, G. R. and Boshuizen, H. P. A. (1990). A cognitive perspective on medical expertise: theory and implications. *Acad. Med.,* **65,** 611–21

10. Raimi, R. A. (1981). Twice told tale — the joy of teaching. *N. Y. Times Spring Survey of Education,* **April 26,** 59

11. Weinberg, A. D., Ullian, L., Richards, W. D. and Cooper, P. (1986). Informal advice and information seeking between physicians. *J. Med. Educ.,* **56,** 174–80

12. Covell, D. G., Uman, G. C. and Manning, P. R. (1985). Information needs in office practice: are they being met? *Ann. Intern. Med.,* **103,** 596–9

13. Haynes, R. B., McKibbon, A., Fitzgerald, D., Guyatt, G. H., Walker, C. J. and Sackett, D. L. (1986). How to keep up with the medical literature: IV. Using the literature to solve clinical problems. *Ann. Intern. Med.,* **105,** 636–40

14. Williamson, J. W., German, P. S., Weiss, R., Skinner, E. A. and Bowes, F. (1989). Health science information management and continuing education of physicians. *Ann. Intern. Med.,* **110,** 151–60

15. Osheroff, J. A. and Bankowitz, R. A. (1993). Physicians' use of computer software in answering clinical questions. *Bull. Med. Libr. Assoc.,* **81,** 11–19

16. Chambliss, M. L. (1992). Personal computer access to Medline: an introduction. *J. Fam. Pract.,* **32,** 414–18

17. Haynes, R. B., McKibbon, K. A., Fitzgerald, D., Guyatt, G. H., Walker, C. J. and Sackett, D. L. (1986). How to keep up with the medical literature: II. Deciding which journals to read regularly. *Ann. Intern. Med.,* **105,** 309–12

18. Albright, R. G. (1988). *A Basic Guide to On-line Information Systems for Health Care Professionals.* (Arlington, VA: Information Resource Press)

19. Siegel, E. R., Cummings, M. M. and Woodsmall, R. M. (1990). Bibliographic-retrieval systems. In Shortliffe, E. H. and Perreault, L. E. (eds.). *Medical Informatics: Computer Applications in Health Care.* (Reading, MA: Addison-Wesley)

20. Haynes, R. B., McKibbon, A., Fitzgerald, D., Guyatt, G. H., Walker, C. J. and Sackett, D. L. (1986). How to keep up with the medical literature: III. Expanding the number of journals you read regularly. *Ann. Intern. Med.,* **105,** 474–8

21. Hoffer, E. P. and Barnett, G. O. (1990). Computers in medical education. In Shortliffe, E. H. and Perreault, L. E. (eds.) *Medical Informatics: Computer Applications in Health Care.* (Reading, MA: Addison-Wesley)

12

Passing the boards

S. Miller and L. D. Victor

INTRODUCTION

There are two moments we will never forget. The day President Kennedy was shot and the day we failed our board examinations. Each was greeted with disbelief, devastation and mourning. We knew we could never change the past. At least with the board examination the future could be different. With hard work and good judgment you can avoid the grief of failure. The following chapter will provide information on how to pass any written board examination. Our experience has been that the qualifying examination for internal medicine certification is among the more difficult, with a 20% failure rate, and so this particular examination will be emphasized.

Passing board examinations is important for your career. Many hospitals require board certification for admitting privileges, and it is generally needed for advancement in academic or teaching environments. Board certification is prestigious; it sends a message to your peers that you are a cut above the rest. The public is also very much aware of board passage. Every day we have patients that have found our name as a board-certified specialist in one of the proprietary listings[1]. Board certification has had financial advantages as well; boarded specialists have historically been compensated better by third-party payers.

Another positive aspect of board examination passage is the perception of others that you can successfully complete a difficult task. Board preparation is similar to preparing for any great event, whether it is in the sporting arena, a wedding, or a public performance. The diligence and single mindedness required for board passage is similar to that shown by Michael Jordan when becoming a great basketball player, or Ghandi when preparing to execute his theories of non-violence. Successful board passage is a message to the doctor as well as his or her peers that they have the capability to succeed in an arduous task. Board examinations are also considered clinically important. In support of this, consider that the average board question is clinically relevant as judged by a panel of primary care practitioners[2].

On the other hand, failure to pass the boards may be perceived as a deficiency in your ability to provide exemplary medical care and can be devastating to your self-confidence and career advancement. Lawyers are also very much aware of the importance of board certification; plaintiffs' attorneys like to ask if you are board certified and how many times it took you to pass. In legal matters, therefore, it can only work to your disadvantage if you have failed a board examination.

Certification boards maintain that their respective exams remain the best indicator of a physican's clinical competence. While board certification is the gold standard in the measurement of clinical knowledge it may not translate into an accurate measure of competency or ethical standards. Board examinations cannot measure honesty, character or compassion, nor do they address what constitutes the art of medicine.

HISTORY OF THE BOARDS

The National Board of Medical Examiners (NBME) was founded in 1915 and initially provided consultative services to the American Board of Pediatrics. The NBME did not become involved in specialty examination until 1961. Prior to this each specialty was responsible for their respective certification exams; the first was the American Board of Ophthalmology (1917). By 1936 ten specialty boards had been created. During the next 2 years, internal medicine (1936) and surgery (1937) incorporated their subspecialty boards. The American Board of Internal Medicine (ABIM) had a somewhat unique vision regarding their views on the purpose of board certification. Whereas other specialties wanted to raise the general level of competence by certifying all physicians, the ABIM had no desire that every practitioner of internal medicine should be board certified. The board-certified internist would be judged as an outstanding consultant, set apart from many of his colleagues in the area of clinical knowledge and competence. Many clinicians still view the internal medicine boards as one of the most difficult examinations.

Subspecialty boards in surgery had already formed before the American Board of Surgery was incorporated in 1937. In 1940, the ABIM decided to certify subspecialists in cardiology, gastroenterology, tuberculosis and allergy, in those physicians already certified in general internal medicine.

Board certification became even more important with the advent of the Second World War[3]. Over 50 000 physicians were members of the armed services. The army could now classify physicians based on their board certification status. Physicians were classified on a scale from A to D with A being the highest. Board certification brought at least a B classification and the ranking of captain. When they returned home, board-certified physicians received higher salaries in specialty residency training and, later on, in their practice with the Veteran's Administration Hospital System.

PREPARING FOR THE BOARDS

Preparation for the boards should begin on the first day of your residency. Every patient you take care of in training will be your textbook. How well you are able to retrieve that data on the day of the examination may determine whether or not you will succeed in passing the boards. The patient with splinter hemorrhages of the nails who had subacute bacterial endocarditis taught you about all the indications for antibiotic prophylaxis of endocarditis. You will never forget the importance of preventative medicine and immunizations after taking care of a patient with tetanus. The opisthotonos noted during the tetanic spasms could never be explained as graphically in a textbook or by a lecturer. The dramatic response of a patient who had cardiac tamponade to a pericardiocentesis helped you understand the physiology behind the physical finding of pulsus paradoxus. Each of these case scenarios could potentially generate dozens of board questions regarding their associated histories, physical findings, diagnosis and treatment. Your residency training experience remains your one greatest resource in your preparation for the boards.

Unfortunately, some residents do not regard their patients as an important source of learning and rely on 2–3 months of intensive studying and attendance of a board review course as adequate preparation for the boards. This is risky behavior. Recent studies by one board has shown a cumulative decline in the test performance of graduates from US medical schools[4].

Maximize your learning

In order to increase your chances of passing your board exam try to maximize your learning experience during your medical school and residency training. We have suggested the following guidelines to assist you.

Approach each patient and their diagnosis as a potential case presentation on the board exam. The data base that you will accumulate from your training experience will be extensive. The trick will be to assimilate and retrieve the data effectively when faced with the same scenario on the boards. List the classic historical and physical examination findings along with roentgenographical and laboratory results and treatment for your patients' diagnoses. The boards usually present typical cases and their associated findings. However, they are also notorious for presenting atypical presentations of common illnesses.

Develop a differential diagnosis list on your patients and consider several other diagnoses that could present in a similar fashion. Include infectious, metabolic, neoplastic, hereditary and endocrine causes of the presenting symptoms. From the textbook of your choice review the chapter on your diagnosis that day.

Know about your patient's treatment efficacy, side effects, medication dosing and cost.

Self-directed, adult learners (see Chapter 11) will consider a brief literature search on your patient's problem. Address any new advancements in the diagnosis and treatment of the disease. As board questions are written well in advance, you may not be able to answer treatment questions based on guidelines established in the few months before administration of your particular examination.

Certain rare diseases will be tested. This is because, when undiagnosed, severe morbidity or mortality can occur. Examples in internal medicine would be Wilson's disease, α_1-antitrypsin deficiency and Addison's disease, etc. Know the currently fashionable diseases well. Do not forget the people writing the exam are also engaged in current research. Scientists worked out all the details of vitamin deficiency in the 1930s. It is unlikely that you will get a case of scurvy on the internal medicine boards, but there will be several questions on AIDS, sleep apnea, Lyme disease and treatment of acute myocardial infarction.

Approach the examination as a learning experience. If you concentrate on areas that you perceive will be useful in practice you will likely be rewarded by questions covering these areas on the exam. The essential body of information from which you will be tested will be practical. Minute detail about the disease processes is not as important as a global understanding. You do not have to get all the answers correct to pass the examination.

Know the basic science of your field. You can expect to see many questions concerning ocular physiology on the ophthalmology boards and radiation physics on the radiology boards. Internists, for example, should know basic cardiac physiology. It would not be unreasonable to expect a candidate to have a fundamental understanding of Starling's law of the heart. The knowledge and application of basic science separates the physician from a physician's assistant.

Know your weaknesses. For example, international medical graduates have many more problems passing boards because of language difficulty. The subtleties of grammar must be understood to answer difficult board questions. International medical graduates may need to study English as well as their specialty information. American graduates that have had difficulty on standardized examinations will almost assuredly have difficulty on certifying board examinations. Those with acknowledged academic weaknesses will have to be particularly driven as they can expect that their board examination will be the most difficult and important examination of their lifetime! Another excellent way to assess your strengths and weaknesses is to ask your program director. One study showed that program director ratings was one of the most important predictors of candidates' board scores[5].

A few study tips
Preparing for board examinations is effective. Studies have shown that experienced test takers who have been coached can do better on standardized examinations[6]. We will now list some important study strategies.

Guard your study time. Set aside a regular time to study and stick to it.

Avoid memorizing material. Board examinations emphasize understanding concepts rather than specific facts.

Talk to recent candidates. It will help you prepare for the board examination if you ask those who have recently taken the exam about the format and general content of the test. While previous examinees are ethically constrained in discussing specific questions there is no problem in telling you about the types of questions and general subject matter. Successful candidates will often share what they feel were their successful preparation and test-taking strategies. Those who failed may provide the most useful information; what did they do wrong?

Board reviews are an effective supplement to preparation. They can identify any weak areas in your medical knowledge base so that you can intensify your studying of those topics. On-going board reviews are probably most effective, as they are continued in a cyclical fashion throughout your entire residency training. Our medicine residency offers three reviews per month in a designated subspecialty of internal medicine. In-training exams (ITE) are also offered by some residency programs to assess the cognitive skills of residents, especially those in the second postgraduate year (PGY-2). In addition to identifying personal areas of deficiency, the residents can compare their performance to that of other residents nationwide. A less than satisfactory performance will alert the resident to inadequate preparation. For example, it has been shown that an empirically derived cut-off score of the 35th percentile on the PGY-2 Internal Medicine In-training Examination had a positive predictive value of 89% (probability of passing the boards) and a negative predictive value of 83% (probability of failing the boards)[7].

How much studying is enough? One does not want to burn out too early. There are rare people who seem to be able to pass exams with a minimum of study time crammed in at the last minute. This technique may have sufficed during college when a good memory often enabled you to pass and survive finals week. Board examinations have a more important function as they are trying to evaluate your clinical judgment. Just studying textbooks will not be enough as board exams attempt to draw off of the candidates real-life experiences. Questions are designed to test the candidate's thorough knowledge and understanding of the disease process in addition to their ability to evaluate and act upon the data presented to them. Anyone can memorize an instruction manual or a textbook. One has to only recall failed attempts at plumbing or electrical repair despite having the home improvement manual in front of you. Nothing takes the place of experience and judgment. Intensive studying, however, can not hurt and may be effective for some people. This is best done sometime during the last year of residency training.

Intensive board reviews: are they useful? Some residents attend these intensive courses which usually last 5 days with 8–10 hours of lectures each day. You are subjected to numerous pearls of wisdom that are guaranteed to show up on the boards. We have mixed feelings about the usefulness of board review courses. If taken a few weeks prior to the exam they may help to bring it all together. On the other hand, they may point out all that you do not know or have forgotten. This can feed into the anxiety and paranoia that will already be substantial. Perhaps the best time to attend a board review would be at the beginning of your intensive study time, about 8–12 months before the examination, so that you could earlier identify your weak areas.

Develop an attitude that you will pass the examination on your first attempt. This is the most useful advice we can provide. Our experience over the years has shown that most successful candidates regard board passage as important from day one of their residency. We see their study intensify as they get into their senior year and closer to the examination. The highly successful candidates regard board passage as a priority over diversions such as football games and partying. Many successful candidates have the support and understanding of their spouse or significant other. Both of you must realize that preparing for the exam is *the* most important priority in each of your lives for the next 6–12 months. Socializing, vacations, moonlighting and recreational activities must all be severely curtailed. In the end you must be able to say to yourself that you did everything you could to prepare for the exam. You do not want to go through this experience again.

DAY OF THE EXAMINATION
The most important thing to remember in your preparation for the boards is that you must be well rested and relaxed on the day of the exam. No one has ever passed the boards because of last minute cramming. Get plenty of sleep. Allow enough time to get to the examination site and remember your registration ticket and personal identification.

Recommendations when taking a board examination

Time limits. During the exam, remember that there may be a time limit that could be strictly enforced throughout the exam for each of the sections. Therefore, it is important that you pace yourself and that you are aware of the time constraints. If you cannot answer a question within a few minutes take an educated guess, record it and move on. There is usually no penalty for a wrong answer so make sure you answer every question. Do not record your answers in the test booklet and then write them on the scoring sheet as you may run out of time before you can rerecord your answers.

Read the questions and answers carefully before answering. For example, are you looking for the one correct answer or the one exception? Another advantage of reading the entire question thoroughly is to improve your ability to capitalize potential test inconsistencies. Every examination the authors have taken has had a tip-off on how to answer an earlier question from another question's statement or answers.

On multiple choice questions eliminate the wrong answers first. Multiple choice questions require you to make true–false decisions on each of the answers[6]. If you have prepared yourself well for the examination there will be few questions that will be totally unfamiliar. Of the four or five possible answers, there are usually one or two ridiculous choices and two or three plausible answers. You can usually hone your answer choices to one or two that you feel may be correct. The answer you choose may not be what you consider ideal, but medical practice is often a matter of opinion. Your only requirement is to pick the best answer.

Watch out for modifiers such as 'all' and 'every'. Absolutes are often seen in mathematics and physics but rarely in medicine.

First hunches tend to be correct. Do not change an answer unless you discover an obvious error or misinterpretation of the question.

General recommendations when taking any test
There are many books available which discuss how to take a test[8–10] — some of the common themes include the following:

(1) Answer all the questions and avoid making stray marks on the answer sheets.

(2) Check your answer sheet often to make sure that you are answering the right questions in the right spot.

(3) During the examination concentrate on answering the questions. Avoid any distractions.

(4) Wear comfortable clothes the day of the exam.

(5) Try to maintain your regular eating and exercise habits just prior to the examination.

(6) Bring sharpened number two pencils and an accurate watch.

IF YOU FAIL THE BOARDS
'The American Board regrets to inform you that you did not pass the certifying exam.' So began the letter that I (Stanley Miller) had anticipated would bring the wonderful news of my board certification. I remember initially feeling numb as I again read the dreadful news. Embarrassment, self-doubt and despair immediately flooded over me. It is amazing, in retrospect, how frail my ego and self-esteem were at that time; mere results of an exam could destroy in seconds what 3 years of residency had proven to myself. What I did in order to pass my boards may well help you pass any difficult examination. The main reasons for my failure to pass the internal medicine boards on my first attempt include four important areas. First, I failed to realize that board passage was the number one priority in my life. Since all other priorities are disrupted because of your board preparation you will not be able to get on with your normal life until you do pass the boards. Do not let anything interfere. One of the authors (Lyle Victor) failed the critical care boards because he edited a medical textbook while studying for the examination.

Second, I (Stanley Miller) was inadequately prepared. I had not started early enough nor accelerated study sufficiently toward the end of my residency. I had to reaffirm my determination to pass the boards and not let my previous failure prevent what had to be done.

Third, I nitpicked. I agonized over knowing the minute details of every disease process; it was not necessary. One must be thorough, but not lose sight of the big picture.

Lastly, I had inadequate study habits. I scheduled inadequate time to study. I should have scheduled all other necessary activities around my designated study time. I should have never compromised this time. In addition, I had an inadequate study environment to foster serious concentration. I should never have studied in front of the television, at the beach or lying down. I should have kept extraneous noise at a minimum and made efforts to avoid unproductive sessions.

SUMMARY
Preparation for board certification is a most serious matter. How badly you want to pass will often determine your success. Our wish for you is that when you one day open up the mail box and remove a letter from your certification board, it reads: 'Congratulations, you have successfully passed the certification exam....'

REFERENCES
1. Anonymous (1993). *Directory of Board Certified Medical Specialists.* (Evanston, IL: Marquis)
2. Norcini, J. J., Day, S. C., Grosso, L. J., Langdon, L. O., Kimball, H. R., Popp, R. L. and Goldfinger, S. E. (1993). The relevance to clinical practice of the Certifying Exam in Internal Medicine. *J. Gen. Intern. Med.*, **8**, 82–5
3. Howell, J. D. (1989). The invention and development of American internal medicine. *J. Gen. Intern. Med.*, **4**, 127–33
4. Norcini, J. J., Shea, J. A. and Benson, J. A. (1991). Changes in the medical knowledge of candidates for certification. *Ann. Intern. Med.*, **114**, 33–5
5. Day, S. C., Grosso, L. J. and Norcini, J. J. (1994). Methods of preparing for the certifying examination in internal medicine and their efficacy. *J. Gen. Intern. Med.*, **9**, 167–9
6. Anastasi, A. (1981). Coaching, test sophistication and developed abilities. *Am. Psychol.*, 1981, **36**, 1086–93
7. Grossman, R. S., Fincher, R. E., Layne, R. D., Seelig, C. B., Berkowitz, L. R. and Levine, M. A. (1992). Validity of the intraining examination for predicting American Board of Internal Medicine Scores. *J. Gen. Intern. Med.*, **7**, 63–7
8. Seibel, H. R. and Guyer, K. (1990). *MCAT How to Prepare for the Medical College Admission Test*, Barrons Educational Series. (New York: Barron)
9. Rudman, J. (1991). *New Rudman's Questions and Answers on the MCAT.* Medical College Admission Test, Admission Test Series. (Syosset, NY: National Learning Corporation)
10. Martinson, T. H. (1988). *Supercourse for the GRE.* (New York: Simon and Schuster)

13

Avoiding lawsuits

D. Craig

INTRODUCTION

You have spent years in preparation for your career in medicine. Although you have some trepidation, you feel confident you have mastered the technical skills and are current on recent advances in medicine. The last thing on your mind is the fear of being sued for medical malpractice. But should you be concerned? The so-called medical malpractice crisis has been on the increase over the last 20 years. The frequency of malpractice claims rose rapidly in the early 1970s, stabilized, then began another upward trend in the early 1980s. Between 1975 and 1985 the number of claims per physician rose at an average rate of 10% per year[1]. As a young physician, your odds are high for becoming another litigation statistic.

Some would argue that the malpractice climate is now worse because the competency of physicians has dramatically decreased over the last 20 years. New advances in medicine would suggest otherwise. Most studies on the cause of increased litigation have concluded that the problem results from a combination of events, primarily the expansive application of tort law, an increasingly complex health care environment and a litigious society[2].

Tremendous advances in medicine have raised expectations for patients who were previously thought to have hopeless or untreatable conditions. Treatment of these conditions, however, is at a price for the physician. New procedures are usually associated with new complications, which may be viewed by patients as negative outcomes.

Tort reform

Meaningful tort reform can have a major impact on stabilizing the professional liability climate, as in Indiana and California. Other states, such as Maine, Texas and Florida, have passed various types of tort reform. Most have some provision for mandatory pretrial screening, expert witness practice and training requirements, limitations on non-economic damages, reductions of statutes of limitations, and sliding scale contingency fees for attorneys representing patients.

In February 1990, Senator Orrin Hatch introduced the 'Ensuring Access to Care through Medical Liability Reform' Act (S.489)[3]. Unfortunately to date, federal legislation has not been forthcoming. Individual states will need to introduce meaningful tort reforms in order to have any impact on the malpractice crisis.

Perceptions

Since meaningful changes in the tort system will be slow in coming, it is important for physicians to take action to address the problem. The first step must be to begin analyzing issues and treatment rendered, from the patient's perspective. Health care professionals and patients have different perceptions of quality care. Physicians view quality in terms of success from a technical standpoint. Was the neurosurgical procedure successful in maintaining the patient's life, although the quality of life may be diminished? Was the orthopedic surgeon able to save the badly crushed limb, even though the patient may need extensive physical therapy and experience pain for the remainder of her life?

Patients and their family members view quality health care in humanistic terms (e.g. caring, supportive, communicative, reliable and empathetic care-givers). Society encourages technological advances, not humanistic characteristics. All things being equal, the patient will see the physician who takes time to explain his disease and options as a better physician than one who does not. A survey conducted by the American Medical Association suggested that the public feels physicians do not care as much about people as they used to, do not spend enough time with their patients, and that they are more motivated by money and prestige than a desire to help people[4].

Communication and caution

Medical school curricula emphasize technical skills, disease processes and treatment modalities. There is little emphasis on communication skills. Medical students learn very early that the technical aspects of their training appear to be more important than developing communication skills.

Can it be assumed that a turn around in medical malpractice litigation could be accomplished if physicians became less detached and more communicative, and patients became more realistic and less demanding of perfectionism? Probably not. We live in a very litigious society. Some patients are prone to sue, regardless of the outcome. Patients who complain about prior physicians, doctor shop (seek care for the same condition from several physicians), are non-compliant, hostile or are seen as malingerers are prone to suing physicians. It is best to act cautiously with these patients, treat them conservatively, keep meticulous records, including missed appointments. If they are not compliant with the treatment plan, consider terminating the physician/patient relationship, after consulting with a legal counsel.

The physician must also realize that she does not only treat the patient, but she treats the family as well. Family perceptions may play a big role in whether a suit is filed. If a physician sees the aforementioned personality traits in family members, she should be just as cautious. Care should be given to maintaining communication with family members, as long as the patient's right to confidentiality is not jeopardized.

High-risk specialties
Even if physicians do not have litigious patients and families by nature, they may be more prone to being sued because of their specialties. Obstetricians/gynecologists, surgical subspecialties (e.g. orthopedic surgeons and neurosurgeons) and emergency medicine physicians have seen a dramatic increase in litigation over the past 10–15 years. Obstetricians have been hit hardest. An American College of Obstetricians and Gynecologists study indicates that an average obstetrician will be sued eight times in a 35-year career[5]. In 1988, it was estimated that a total of 73% of practicing obstetricians in the US had been sued; 40% had been sued three or more times[6].

Why are obstetricians, orthopedic surgeons, neurosurgeons and emergency medicine physicians more prone to being sued? It is thought by some that these specialties have a higher probability of producing adverse outcomes in the absence of error. If errors are made they are more detectable and can result in more severely injured patients than in most other areas of medical practice[7].

Resident physicians practicing in certain specialties are also more prone to being sued. A study conducted by the Risk Management Foundation of the Harvard Medical Institution found that nearly 75% of malpractice cases involving resident physicians originated in surgical specialties[8]. The emergency department was the most likely department for an incident to occur. One third of all malpractice cases that occur in the emergency department name resident physicians as defendants, which has obvious implications for those who moonlight. Resident physicians are particularly vulnerable because they do not possess all the skills and experience that comes with time. It is therefore necessary for resident physicians to carefully evaluate the pros and cons of moonlighting.

PREVENTIVE MEASURES

Know where allegations are made
In the event a physician is sued, he will be charged with specific allegations of medical malpractice. The most common allegations are:

(1) Failure to treat/failure to diagnose;

(2) Failure to obtain timely consultations;

(3) Miscommunication or improper communication between health care providers;

(4) Unnecessary treatment;

(5) Negligent or improper treatment;

(6) Failure to respond;

(7) Premature discharge;

(8) Failure to obtain consent;

(9) Equipment malfunction; and

(10) Abandonment.

Many lawsuits include a combination of the aforementioned allegations. Each of these will now be discussed in turn.

Failure to diagnose a patient's condition. This can result from a number of causes. Generally, it is not due to a physician's inadequate knowledge base, but rather due to a miscommunication between hospital departments (laboratory, radiology or emergency department) which leads to an adverse outcome for the patient.

Failure to diagnose a condition may also stem from the physician's inappropriate sense of overconfidence, particularly if he has heard the same symptoms from hundreds of patients before. The physician must remember that each patient is unique and requires the same thorough history and physical examination. Even if the physician feels that he knows what the problem is, he or she should order the appropriate tests to confirm his or her suspicions. In most cases the suspicions will be borne out. But in some cases they will not, and additional tests and investigation will be necessary.

Failure to obtain the appropriate consultants at the right time. Generally, consultants are not requested for egotistical reasons — the physician does not want to admit to himself, the patient or family that the patient's condition is beyond his training and expertise. Physicians unwilling to bring in consultants often pay a high price for it. It is very important to put the patient's condition before your ego. Remember, the practice of medicine has become very complex. Specialists are trained to assist in the care of the patient suffering from complex medical conditions. Take advantage of their skills.

Miscommunication or improper communication between health care professionals. Miscommunication often gives rise to litigation and this is usually seen when hospital departments fail to communicate needed information to the physician. It is most evident in the emergency department. Findings on X-ray or laboratory test results may not be communicated to the emergency department physician in a timely manner. As a result, patients may be discharged from the emergency department before abnormal results have been received. It is imperative that physicians be aware of all tests and procedures ordered, and obtain the results before discharging patients.

Improper communication also occurs when a nurse, physician or other health care providers make negative comments to the patient regarding his treatment. Comments made by uninformed people can be detrimental, especially if they recommend another course of treatment. These criticisms, whether intentional or not, undermine the patient/ physician relationship and must be avoided, as they can lead to a lawsuit.

Negligent or improper treatment. Unnecessary treatment often stems from a physician's failure to properly take a thorough history and physical, and request the right consultants. As a result, a physician may undertake a course of treatment that may not be justified because the investigations were inadequate. Unnecessary treatment may also stem from improper judgment or inadequate technical skills.

Physician's failure to respond. This is another common allegation which relates particularly to surgical specialties, especially obstetrics. With some surgical and obstetrical conditions, time is of the essence. The patient should expect her physician to respond within a certain time when needed. It is important that every physician has a back-up system so that patients' needs can be addressed in a timely manner. For sole practitioners, this can be a particular problem if prior arrangements for coverage have not been made with other physicians. A suit may be brought on this basis, if an answering service, hospital operator, nursing supervisor or the patient herself cannot contact a physician when needed. It is important that all appropriate people are notified of any substitutions in coverage.

In obstetrics, a timely response may be crucial to the patient's ultimate outcome. The obstetrician must remain in contact with the nursing staff to determine the patient's progress, if he or she is unable to be present to observe it. It is also imperative that the obstetrician gives strict parameters on when to be called. If an emergency Cesarean section is required, the obstetrician must be able to respond within minutes.

Premature discharge. With the pressure peer review organizations are placing on physicians to discharge patients, some litigation is being seen as a result of premature discharge. The physician's medical judgment should never give way to financial considerations if the care of the patient requires a longer hospitalization. The physician is ultimately responsible for the care of the patient, and should use good medical judgment when discharging patients.

Failure to obtain consent. Many lawsuits allege that the patient received inadequate or incomplete information before undergoing a procedure or surgery, and as a result the patient did not give informed consent. In order to protect yourself from this allegation the physician should have a thorough discussion with the patient, and/or his or her family or legal guardian if appropriate, regarding the patient's condition, diagnosis and prognosis. Also, the risks and benefits of the proposed treatment or procedure, and the risks and benefits of alternative treatments or procedures, including no treatment at all, should be discussed. The patient should be given every opportunity to ask questions and have a thorough understanding before consenting to treatment.

Equipment malfunction. Another allegation commonly seen in professional liability cases is the malfunctioning or failure of equipment. Although most of the equipment used at a hospital is maintained by the hospital, there may be times when the physician is responsible for its control and functioning. Whenever possible, the physician should test any equipment he or she will be using (e.g. cautery or suctioning devices) prior to its use on a patient.

Abandonment. Finally, an emerging cause of action is the abandonment of the patient which detrimentally affects the patient's health. This usually arises when there has been a breakdown in the physician/patient relationship. If a breakdown in the relationship occurs, then the physician should discuss the problem with the patient, if this is at all possible. When problems cannot be resolved, the patient should be treated by another physician. The initial physician should not withdraw from the case until another physician has accepted the patient. If a physician is dealing with a difficult patient, she may wish to terminate the physician/patient relationship, but this must be done in such a way as not to jeopardize the patient's health. Legal guidance should be sought prior to terminating a relationship with the patient.

Maintaining good relationships
In addition to being alert to the most common allegations brought against physicians, you can minimize the chances of being sued by simply maintaining good human relation skills. A good rapport with the patient and family will go a long way in avoiding a lawsuit.

Dorothy Rasinski, MD, JD, has outlined the nine Rs of malpractice prevention[9]. They include:

(1) *Rapport:* establish good relationships with patients, their relations, and hospital and office staff;

(2) *Rationale:* use an acceptable plan of diagnosis and treatment;

(3) *Records:* document the performance of the plan;

(4) *Remarks:* avoid offhand, gratuitous and 'silent comments';

(5) *RXs:* register contraindications, interactions and allergies to drugs;

(6) *Res ipsa loquitur:* if the matter speaks for itself, make prompt and adequate restitution;

(7) *Respect:* show respect for the patient's wishes, background and culture;

(8) *Results:* itemize the possibilities in advance, both good and bad;

(9) *Risks:* discuss risks fully before obtaining the patient's consent.

Good human relation skills should be used, beginning with the initial contact with the patient and/or the family. Introducing yourself as Dr Smith and calling the patient by Mr, Mrs or Miss until told otherwise, demonstrates respect for the patient. When taking a patient's history, try to be at eye level with the patient. Again this conveys concern and respect.

Taking a patient's history is very important, but it is usually viewed as a time-consuming task. During the history, the patient conveys his subjective feelings and symptoms, which may be key in making a diagnosis. The physician must *listen* intently. It does a disservice to the patient and can be dangerous for the physician to have a preconceived notion of the patient's problem and therefore fail to hear key information. Many a lawsuit has been generated because of an incomplete history and physical, resulting in the obvious being found but the subtle overlooked. Although documentation will be discussed in more detail later, it is important that you document the patient's history very carefully and thoroughly.

Following a complete history, the patient should undergo a physical examination. This may be stressful or even painful for the patient, and should be done in such a way so as to minimize these factors. As you examine the patient it is important to ask questions and observe the patient's responses, both verbal and non-verbal. Following your examination, ask the patient if she has any other information or questions she wishes to convey to you. Even if the patient does not ask any questions, the physician should always provide the patient with a plan for the hospitalization (e.g. diagnostic tests and consultations, etc.). The amount of information shared with the patient will depend on the patient's mental and physical status and the medical condition being treated. Again it is necessary to document your physical findings in detail. If you follow this routine, you will leave the patient with a positive impression of a concerned, knowledgeable and competent physician.

Good documentation

The outcome of many lawsuits depends on the quality of the documentation in the medical record. Following a few simple rules, you will be more successful in establishing a record that can be used to defend you in the case of litigation.

(1) Document abnormal and significant normal findings of the patient;

(2) Document your thought process and rationale for the care rendered and rationale for omitting or delaying certain tests;

(3) Document and review conversations with others (physicians, patients or family members);

(4) Document your awareness of any problems and your follow-up to them; and

(5) Correct inappropriate entries in the proper manner.

These five recommendations, although seemingly oversimplified, are very important. Always remember, the time spent in documenting will save you 10-fold the time needed to defend a lawsuit (meeting with attorneys, depositions and trial, etc.). I will now discuss the significant matters relating to documentation.

Abnormal and significant normal findings. Beginning with the history and physical, the physician must document abnormal findings and significant normal findings. Even if a finding is normal, it may be significant to the patient's overall condition. For example, a patient may have a history of migraine headaches, but now presents with leg weakness. If a thorough neurological examination is documented with normal and abnormal findings, this should include the fact that the patient is not currently complaining of a headache. It is a significant normal finding which may prove to be crucial to the investigations or treatment plan. It is also important to document a significant history, such as alcoholism, venereal disease or previous abortion, even if it may be embarrassing to the patient. Certain information may be pertinent to other physicians and so they must have knowledge of that information.

Your best defense. The medical record is usually the only tangible piece of evidence the physician has available to defend himself if sued. A general principle is, if it was not documented, it is presumed that it was not performed. If a physician poorly documents, his credibility may be questioned if he tries to defend himself years later at the time of trial. It is best to think of the medical record as a written story of the patient's hospitalization and, therefore, should read like a book. If the record does not flow, it is quite possible that key information has been left out.

The record should reflect your thought processes. The rationale for ordering tests and consultations should be documented. More importantly, if tests are not going to be ordered, the record should reflect the reasons for not ordering the test. This documentation eliminates any second guessing of your care, provided your decisions were based on sound medical judgment.

Relevant conversations. Any time there is a conversation that is relevant to the patient's care, whether with a physician, nurse, family member or the patient himself, it should be documented in the record, even pertinent telephone conversations. All documentation should be in a factual and objective manner, and the chart should never be used as a battling ground between professionals or as an editorial page. Disputes between health care providers should be resolved outside the view of others (patients, family members and other health care providers), and according to the appropriate chain of command, if necessary.

Other health care workers' records. In addition to good documentation, it is also important that the physician reviews other health care providers' documentation, especially that of consultants and nurses. Nurses are more apt to document subtle changes in the patient, which gives you information about the previous 24 hours. Also review consultants' notes. If they recommend a course of treatment, follow it up. If you disagree with the recommendations, make sure your documentation reflects your rationale and justification for your present course of treatment.

Awareness of change and your response. Your documentation should also demonstrate your awareness of any problem or change in the patient's condition, and your response to it. When a patient's medical condition changes, document your awareness of it, make a decision as to necessary follow up (additional tests or O_2, etc.), write the orders, and document your rationale and thought process for doing so. Often a patient's condition changes, but there is nothing medically that can be done about it. Your notes should, however, reflect your awareness of the problem and that no intervention need be, or can be, taken at that time.

Correction of documentation. Another rule of thumb in documentation is if an error in charting is made (e.g. wrong patients' chart or inaccurate information), it should be corrected promptly and properly. Do not obliterate the entry. Simply put a single line through the entry, date, time and initial it. Place an explanation above the entry such as 'wrong patient's chart,' or simply put the correct information in the chart. Never write 'error,' because this denotes that something was done improperly.

Communication and the patient's privacy. In addition to appropriate and thorough documentation, the physician must also remember that it is necessary to have good communication skills with family members. Communication with family members must be balanced against the patient's right of privacy. It is helpful to have a discussion with the patient on whether he objects to discussing his care with family members. If the patient objects, the family should be treated courteously and communicated information subject to the limitations the patient has requested.

Clear discharge notes. Another tool in avoiding litigation is to provide clear discharge instructions, particularly in the emergency department.

Merely a note indicating 'discharge instructions given' is not sufficient, the doctor should provide documented instructions (e.g. 'change dressing and apply bacitracin three times per day, return to office for suture removal in 7 days,' etc.). If booklets or form sheets are provided to the patient, they should contain enough information so as to provide the patient with adequate instructions. It is also helpful to have the patient indicate by his signature that he received discharge instructions.

When any discharge instructions are given, it is important that they are given to the patient, both verbally and in writing, in terms that he can understand. The physician should be careful not to use medical terminology or abbreviations when providing instructions to the patient. Medical terminology and abbreviations are appropriate in the medical record, but are not appropriate when conveying information to a lay person.

Dealing with problem patients

Even though armed with sufficient tools to handle most situations, not all patients are easy to communicate with, nor do they always follow medical instructions.

Non-compliance. When patients are non-compliant, your awareness of this should be discussed with the patient at the earliest opportunity. It may be that the patient is non-compliant because your plan of treatment is not consistent with his lifestyle. For patients in need of physical therapy, the lack of transportation can create a big obstacle. If this is the case, physical therapy at home, other transportation options, or closer physical therapy centers may be preferable options for the patient. A patient may experience a side effect of a drug, and thinking there are no alternative medications, decide to stop the medication rather than tolerate a side effect. Changing a patient's medication may resolve the non-compliance.

Patients who are truly non-compliant pose a real risk for litigation. To protect yourself, all conversations and instructions should be carefully documented. If the patient is to return in 3 weeks, make the appointment before the patient leaves, and give him or her an appointment card. Document these steps in the medical record. If a test needs to be done, make the arrangements and give any preparatory instructions to the patient. Again, document this in the medical record. All old appointment books should also be kept. An appointment canceled by the patient should not be erased out of the appointment book; simply document 'no show' or 'canceled by patient' next to the patient's name.

If the patient continues to be non-compliant, the physician may need to take steps to sever the physician/patient relationship. Great care should, however, be taken to avoid a claim of abandonment. Legal advice should be sought before proceeding. A letter to the patient outlining the facts, which demonstrates his non-compliance and the implications of not complying with your treatment plan, should be sent. If the patient's non-compliance may jeopardize his health or life, such opinions should be spelled out. The physician should be careful to use terms easily understood by the patient.

Patients who leave against medical advice. Documentation is again important. A patient wishing to leave against medical advice should never be discharged by evidence of a physician's discharge order. This implies that the physician agrees with the patient's decision to leave the hospital. If a patient wishes to leave against medical advice, and is competent, a long discussion of the risks and implications of leaving should be held with the patient. The implications should be stated in very simple and forthright terms. This discussion, with specifics, should be documented in the chart.

Dealing with problem health care workers
In addition to problem patients, there are problem physicians and other health care workers who may increase your risk of litigation, including individuals who are substance abusers, incompetent, have poor bedside manners or lack insurance coverage. These workers should be avoided if possible. Obtain consultations from others or minimize your involvement with these people. When appropriate, these individuals should be encouraged to seek help.

LITIGATION STRESS SYNDROME
Even if all the advice in this chapter is incorporated into your practice, you may still be sued. If this occurs you can take steps to make it easier on yourself, your family and patients. Being sued invokes a major emotional response. Initially there is anger and disbelief. Any warmth or understanding the physician may have had for the patient is gone.

Studies performed by Dr Sara Charles, a psychiatrist at the University of Illinois at Chicago, found that nearly 40% of physicians experience a major depressive disorder related to professional liability risk exposure[10]. Besides anger, physicians may experience a depressed mood, inner tension, frustration, instability, insomnia, fatigue, gastro-intestinal symptoms, headache, difficulty concentrating, diminished appetite and reduced sex drive[11]. The accumulation of these symptoms in response to being sued has become known as the litigation stress syndrome[12].

Five stages of litigation stress syndrome have been described[13].

(1) *Denial:* how can this be happening to me?

(2) *Anger:* how dare they charge me with malpractice?

(3) *Bargaining:* if I survive this, I promise to be an even better health care provider in the future.

(4) *Depression:* I am in a hopeless situation and it will only get worse.

(5) *Acceptance:* I can only cope with the situation as best I can, and then I will recover.

It is important for the physician to share feelings with others, such as a significant other person, friends or colleagues. Support groups are also very helpful in better understanding and dealing with issues and improving coping skills. A specially trained facilitator (social worker, psychologist or psychiatrist) may be helpful in getting the group to discuss pertinent issues.

Being involved in a support group does not necessarily allow the physician to go forth and practice medicine unscathed. Any physician who has had the unfortunate experience of being sued will always look at his patients differently, practice more cautiously, and may even give up some or all of his practice as a response. The practice of medicine will never again be the same for that physician.

To avoid the unpleasant experience of being sued, the physician should take the necessary precautions outlined in this chapter. As Dorothy Rasinski, MD, JD, the author of the Rs of malpractice prevention, has simply put it: 'Practice the best medicine at all times; treat the patient with care, concern, humanness and respect; and prepare and maintain careful records.'[9]

REFERENCES

1. Danzon, P. M. (1986). The frequency and severity of medical malpractice claims: new evidence. *Law Contemp. Probl.*, **49**, 57–84
2. Spencer, F. C. and Halley, M. M. (1990). The harmful effects of the 'bad doctor' myth. *Bull. Am. Coll. Surg.*, **75**, 6–12
3. Hatch, O. (1991). Ensuring access through medical liability reform act (S.489), 102nd Congress, 1st Session. In *137 Congress Recordings S.* 2324–32
4. Freshnock, L. (1984). Physician and public opinion on health care issues: 1984. In *Survey and Opinion Research.* (Chicago: American Medical Association)
5. Anonymous (1986). *Litigation Assistant: A Guide for the Defendant Physician.* (Washington DC: American College of Obstetrics and Gynecology)
6. Pearse, W. H. (1988). Professional liability: epidemiology and demography. *Clin. Obstet. Gynecol.*, **31**, 148
7. Jacobson, P. D. (1989). Medical malpractice and the tort system. *J. Am. Med. Assoc.*, **262**, 3320–7
8. Shulkin, D. J. (1990). Resident forum, potential liability problems. *J. Am. Med. Assoc.*, **264**, 24
9. Rasinski, D. (1982). Risk management in practice. *Internist*, **23**, 12–20
10. Charles, S. C. (1991). The psychological trauma of a medical malpractice suit: a practical guide. *Am. Coll. Surg. Bull.*, **76**, 22–6
11. Barber, H. R. K. (1991). The malpractice crisis in obstetrics and gynecology: is there a solution? *Bull. N. Y. Acad. Med.*, **67**, 162–72
12. Youngberg, B. J. and Soto, C. (1990). Litigation stress support groups for health care professionals: risk manager's role. *Perspect. Healthcare Risk Management*, **10**, 14–17
13. Patrick, G. B. (1988). Small deaths: an editorial. *ACMS Bull.*, **x**, 1303–6

14

Financial planning for the resident

D. A. Victor

INTRODUCTION

Your many years of hard work are about to pay off. Professionally, you will be given greater responsibilities and allowed to concentrate on facets of medicine that most interest you. Financially, you will be earning a modest salary, perhaps enough to avoid sinking even deeper into debt, but probably not enough to get ahead. And just over the horizon? Much greater financial rewards, you hope.

But at what cost? By the time you enter your specialty, you will have expended many of your most productive years pursuing academic goals, using up financial resources that you have not yet earned, while others have been out in the real world, earning a living. This means that after your residency you must make up for lost time. But physicians are notorious for their poor business sense and even poorer judgment regarding their personal finances.

If you are like others, you might attempt to turn your financial decisions over to 'the professionals' while you pursue the more noble role of a healer. At some future point you will inevitably learn the hard way that others do not always have your best interest in mind, or are simply unlucky or incompetent. It is important to know when to seek the counsel of others and when to rely on your own. This begins by getting past the myth that you are incapable of understanding your own finances as well as the so-called experts, such as certain accountants, attorneys, insurance people and stockbrokers calling themselves estate planners and investment advisers. Once they extend themselves beyond their own area of training, they will make bad investment decisions like everyone else.

You should view the management of your finances as a part of your coming of age — something that adults *must* do for themselves. Budgeting, balancing a checkbook, deciding what you can afford, what you cannot afford, planning for long-term financial goals; these are tasks like shopping for groceries or tying your own shoe laces, sometimes mundane, not always pleasant or fun, but necessary just the same. The sad truth is that when it comes to finances, most adults remain perpetually adolescent.

Years ago I had a friend who purchased a Mercedes just after moving into a new expensive Californian condominium.

> 'Very impressive,' I said, 'you must be doing well.'
> 'I guess so,' he responded, sounding rather vague.
> 'You don't know? How could you *not* know?'
> 'Well,' he said, "the deal was that the condo was for my wife, the car was for me. My accountant figured it out and told me that I could afford both.'

Some quick calculations on his part would have revealed that he could afford neither. My friend was hearing what he wanted to hear. It is these types of immature attitudes toward money that lead to disaster. And, by the way, when they settled their divorce, she got both the house and the proceeds from the sale of the car.

Your residency might be the first true paying position, other than seasonal or part-time jobs. It is a hiatus between the academic world and the business world. And it is an ideal time to develop sound financial principles and habits for the future. Seize this opportunity, because once you are beyond these next few years, life will never be quite as simple again.

YOUR LIFE CYCLE

Your life sequence — school, job, marriage, child-rearing, back to being a couple as children leave the nest, back to being alone as one spouse dies — will be very similar for everyone (Figure 14-1). Typically, the cost sequence proceeds as follows: costs are lower during the brief period before children become part of the family; costs rise as children are born and grow up, and peak during their high school and college years; and as children become adults and leave the household, family costs begin to decline[1].

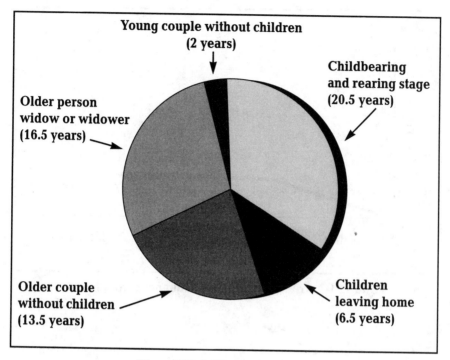

Young couple without children
(2 years)

Childbearing
and rearing stage
(20.5 years)

Older person
widow or widower
(16.5 years)

Older couple
without children
(13.5 years)

Children
leaving home
(6.5 years)

Figure 14-1. Family life cycle

Every household will have a view of its long-term income or *lifetime income.* For example, students who are training to become doctors have a very different view of expected lifetime income than those who are training to become schoolteachers, or assembly line workers, or professional athletes[2]. Because of the expense and duration of your training, your income life sequence will vary quite substantially from the norm. The traditional family income cycle (Figure 14-2) goes like this: income rises gradually from young adulthood through the child-rearing years, remains relatively stable from the middle years until retirement, then stays fixed or actually declines after semi-retirement and retirement[3].

Your monetary cycle will probably proceed as follows: a net loss of income until your training is complete, income rises precipitously just after your residency and slows to regular but healthy yearly increases throughout your child-rearing years, then stays fixed or declines after semi-retirement and retirement (Figure 14-3).

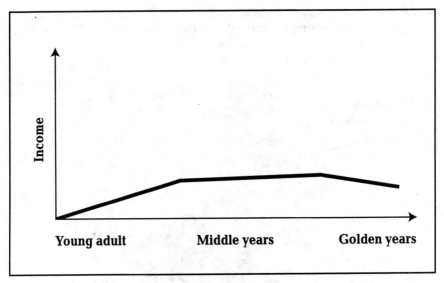

Figure 14-2. Traditional income sequence through life

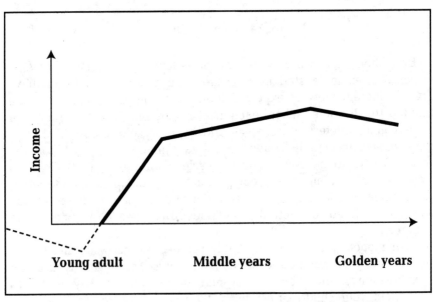

Figure 14-3. Your probable income sequence through life

Ultimately, like everyone else, you will have to face a changing concept of retirement in our nation. Medicine will have the ever-increasing and costly capacity of keeping people alive longer. And what will the AIDS epidemic eventually cost? What will be the result of decades of profligate spending by government, and the eroding work ethic of our citizens? And the cost of letting our educational system decay? Will Social Security be there as a safety net?

Baby-boomers will first enrich, then deplete the nation's retirement system. They will require homes that, later, will have no eager buyers. Ultimately they will require medical care which, if they fail to provide for it, may be denied them. One result of all these things is almost a certainty; most people will have to work, at least part-time, long past the traditional age of retirement[4].

SETTING GOALS

It has been said that if all our nation's wealth was gathered together, then divided evenly among the citizenry, within a week there would once again be rich people and poor people. This hyperbole contains enough grain of truth to strike a chord. For most people, financial goals are immediate, shaped by impulsive habits. Financial success throughout your life cycle will depend upon breaking from this kind of behavior, formulating sensible short- and long-term goals, and well-planned asset management.

During your residency the short-term objective of just stretching your paycheck so that it will cover month-to-month expenses will probably be your main concern. It is for this very reason that you need to plan more carefully than someone of greater affluence, because every dollar will mean that much more to you. It is never too early to start forming notions regarding such concepts as retirement income, estate planning, investment planning and college funds for your children. And now is definitely the time to learn how to assess and monitor your financial status, budget your resources, and resist impulsive purchases.

Here are some important objectives for the formative and middle years:

Ages 18–30:

(1) Train for your career;

(2) Begin to identify long-term goals;

(3) Purchase modest amounts of insurance according to needs;

(4) Develop prudent attitudes toward credit and finances; and

(5) Write a will.

Ages 30–45:

(1) Purchase your own home and establish a permanent household;

(2) Attain financial independence and pay off school loans;

(3) Start a savings program;

(4) Establish a credit identity;

(5) Start an investment program;

(6) Provide for child-rearing and education;

(7) Expand career goals;

(8) Expand insurance according to needs; and

(9) Review and change your will according to needs.

A major change in the last two decades is the substantial increase in one-person, and two-wage-earner households. If you live alone, then there should be extra funds available at the end of each month for savings. This should also be true if there are two persons and an extra paycheck to help with expenses. Forget extra savings for now if there are children in the picture; they are expensive to have, and even more expensive to raise.

If you are married, it is important that you and your spouse have similar attitudes and objectives. Issues of finance are a major cause of marital friction. You should sit down with your spouse, come to a meeting of minds and work out a philosophy.

YOUR FINANCIAL PLAN
A formally devised financial plan is a written blueprint. Its development involves the systematic interrelation of insurance, estate, retirement

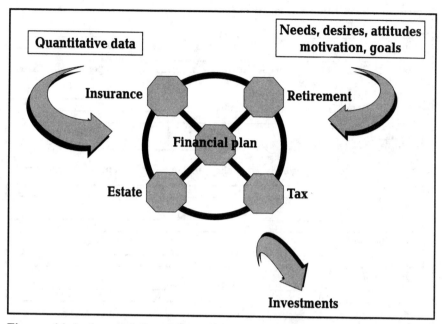

Figure 14-4. A good financial plan will involve the systematic inter-relation of insurance, estate, retirement and tax planning. Examination of these plans will help in the selection of the most appropriate investments

and tax planning. An orderly process of plan development, as shown in Figure 14-4, allows an immediate examination of all financial areas so that you can consider and select the most appropriate investments[5].

There will be many vague areas or voids in your plan because of limited resources and the fact that you are just starting out. For instance, the extent of your estate planning might be the execution of a simple will, and your investment strategy might be as simple as harboring modest sums of money in a money market account until they are needed. In fact, except for certain aspects related to the gathering and analysis of data, it need not be a formally written document at this point, cast in concrete, but simply an overall, inchoate philosophy that changes as your life changes. Its main function, now, is to bring orderliness into your life so that you can have the luxury of feeling that you are in control, and are not simply being swept along with events.

Family Members
Name _____ Birth date _____ S.S. number _____
Name _____ Birth date _____ S.S. number _____
Name _____ Birth date _____ S.S. number _____
Name _____ Birth date _____ S.S. number _____

Wills
Husband – Date _____ Executor _____
Wife   – Date _____ Executor _____
Location of originals _____

Insurance
Life insurance – location of policies _____
Summary:

	Insurer	Insured	Policy number	Amount	Beneficiary

Disability
Insurer _____ Policy number _____
Location _____
Automobile
Insurer _____ Policy number _____
Location _____
Homeowner's
Insurer _____ Policy number _____
Location _____

Bank Accounts
Bank _____ Account number _____
Bank _____ Account number _____

Money Market Account, Stocks and Bonds
Brokerage _____ Account number _____
Stocks   Bonds

_____   _____
_____   _____

Mutual funds
Fund _____ Account number _____
Fund _____ Account number _____
Other investments
Description & location of documents _____

Credit Cards
Issuer _____ Number _____
Issuer _____ Number _____

School loans
Lender & location of document _____

Tax Records – Location _____

Financial Advisors

	Name	Address	Phone
Lawyer			
Broker			
Insurance agent			
Other			

Figure 14-5. The financial review form

GETTING STARTED

Your philosophy will begin taking shape as you collect financial information similar to that shown in Figure 14-5. Once completed, this information should be stored in a file cabinet with other important documents, so that it is always simple to locate. Other irreplaceable papers and valuables should be kept in a safety deposit box (Table 14-1). As a resident, your mind will be cluttered with a thousand-and-one things to remember, and items kept in dresser drawers or cupboards are easily lost. An added note — a *copy* of your will, not the original, should be kept in the safety deposit box, because some states require that the box be sealed immediately following the holder's death, and only opened after the will is read.

Table 14-1. Places to keep valuables and important documents

File drawer	Safety deposit box
Financial review forms	Birth certificates
Paid receipts	Marriage certificates
filed under headings	Leases
Unpaid receipts	Wills (copies)
filed under headings	Citizenship papers
Canceled checks	Divorce decree
Bank statements	Passport
Tax receipts, returns	Bonds, stock certificates
Employment records	Auto titles
Health benefit information	List — household valuables
Insurance policies	Video — household valuables
Wills (originals)	Adoption papers
Family health records	Veteran's papers
Warranties/manuals	Death certificates
School transcripts	Contracts
Safe deposit inventory	Heirlooms, rare/gold coins and
	stamps, etc.

The two review forms that are most helpful to your financial self-analysis are the balance sheet and the budget statement.

The balance sheet in Figure 14-6 demonstrates a financial condition at a particular point in time. It is similar to a single frame of a motion picture. A series of balance sheets over time will give you a moving picture of a

Dr Jones
January 1, 19___

Assets			Liabilities and net worth	
Cash and cash equivalents:			*Liabilities:*	
Checking account	$	1 200	Mortgage balance	$ 100 000
Savings account		3 600	Auto loan balance	5 000
Money market		25 000	Credit cards	1 200
Cash		550		
			Total liabilities	**$ 106 200**
Total	$	30 350		
			Net worth = Assets – Liabilities	
Invested assets:				
Whole life cash value	$	10 000	**Net worth**	**$ 604 150**
Stocks		65 000		
Bonds		50 000		
Vested pension plan		70 000		
Vested profit sharing		85 000		
Total		$ 280 000		
Use assets:				
Residence		$ 250 000		
Automobiles		20 000		
Personal articles		85 000		
Furnishings		45 000		
Total		$ 400 000		
Total asssets		**$ 710 350**		

Figure 14-6. The balance sheet

changing financial condition. As you can see, it is quite simple. On one side are assets divided up into those that are highly liquid, and those that are not. A highly liquid asset is one that can be converted into cash almost immediately, while those listed as use assets must be assigned an estimated market value. You should be most conservative in estimating personal articles and furnishings, because they tend to lose value the quickest after purchase and are the most difficult to convert to cash.

Assets are offset on the right side of the page by liabilities or debts. Your net worth will be what is left after deducting liabilities from assets. Do not be too disappointed if your student loans have created a negative net worth because you are just starting out. However, if the same is true when you are in your forties, seek professional help because you are in trouble.

A budget — people are constantly in the position of having 'too much month at the end of their money.' They ask, 'where does all the money go?' And they rarely are interested in an answer if they are addicted to 'things,' because they just might find out that they cannot afford their lifestyle. A family budget will quickly answer this question. It is a business plan for your household, estimating future expenditures based upon your anticipated income, then comparing these figures with the actual ones. If followed, it will insure that the household will make wise spending decisions so that your constantly changing net worth will change in the right direction.

The secret to success here is flexibility. If you become too complex and elaborate in your record keeping, unwilling to deviate every once in a while, your family will quickly rebel and lose interest. Remember, a budget is not just for people who cannot handle money, and it should not be taken as a form of punishment. My suggestion is to follow a written budget closely for a predetermined time period, just until you have established spending guidelines and patterns.

There are two good ways to accomplish this. You can keep a record of monthly income and living expenses (Figure 14-7) for approximately 3–6 months, so that you can readily see the sources of your income (salary and interest for example), identify fixed and important expenses, and see how much goes for non-essentials. You will then get an idea of what you can save each month. Most people use much more of their income on meaningless non-essentials than they realize. If this type of spending is carefully controlled, it is not unreasonable to expect a modest savings rate of 10–15%. Your first goal with these savings is to establish an emergency fund. It should eventually amount to 6 months take-home pay to provide a cushion in case you should find yourself unemployed.

Another approach is to keep a personal financial diary: looking back without looking ahead. There are a multitude of tiny expenditures, from chewing gum, candy bars and soft drinks, to news-stand magazines and newspapers. This technique will prove effective if you constantly find yourself in the position of having $40 in your pocket on Monday and $2 on Friday, and no recollection of what happened in between. Simply record faithfully, and without exception, every single penny you spend. Do this for a month and you will have a clear picture of where the money goes[6].

Now is a good time to decide whether credit cards are really necessary. Visa and MasterCard are very convenient, and provide a helpful record of expenditures. I would suggest, however, that they are inappropriate until you have an emergency reserve set aside. If you do not heed this advice,

Income	Anticipated	Actual
Wages		
Interest		
Dividends		
Bonus or commission		
Other		
Total Income		
Expenses		
Mortgage		
Rent		
Household maintenance and repairs		
Food		
Electric		
Gas (heating)		
Garbage collection		
Water		
Clothing		
Personal care		
Medications		
Dentist		
Doctor		
Optician		
Oil		
Telephone		
Car loan		
Car maintenance		
Gas (car)		
Car insurance		
Parking		
Public transportation		
Homeowners' insurance		
Life insurance		
Disability insurance		
Child care		
Taxes		
Charitable contributions		
Furniture		
Recreation		
Meals out		
Vacation		
Gifts		
Other		
Total expenses		
Total income minus total expenses		

Figure 14-7. The monthly budget

and find that you are unable to pay off the balance on your credit cards each month, resulting in high finance charges, then destroy all of your credit cards without delay.

In summary, the development of a good financial plan begins with the following three processes:

(1) Identifying important goals and objectives;

(2) Collecting and organizing financial information; and

(3) Drawing up a balance sheet and using a budget to keep track of expenditures.

Now you are ready to address the areas of insurance, estate, retirement and tax planning.

RISK MANAGEMENT (INSURANCE)

There is more to risk management than the purchase of an insurance policy. It involves all of the possible methods for handling the uncertainty of loss. The objective here is to avoid economic loss, and more important, minimize emotional stress. There are three general types of risk that confront us:

(1) Personal risks affecting life and health;

(2) Property risks leading to personal damage or loss; and

(3) Liability risks resulting in the injury or property loss of others.

Risk management involves the use of common sense, and will include all of the methods of treating risks, such as loss prevention, avoidance, self-insurance and risk transfer.

Loss prevention and reduction is a sensible approach that mitigates hazards before they become perils. Covering a slippery floor and fixing faulty electrical wiring would fall within this category. Risk avoidance might involve driving less, or avoiding dangerous sports, or even avoiding moonlighting jobs to supplement your income so that you can always function better as a resident.

Self-insurance is the act of personally assuming a risk of loss, either totally or in varying degrees. People selling insurance will want you to buy as much coverage as possible. Obviously insuring trivial day-to-day losses is unnecessary. In fact, assuming more risk by increasing the amount of time you must wait to collect on a disability policy could significantly reduce the premium. The degree of self-insurance should be based upon how large a loss you can sustain without suffering hardship.

Risk transfer relieves one party of the burden of risk and transfers it to another. This is the purpose of various forms of insurance. As a resident you will probably have to consider four types: disability, automobile, life and homeowners.

Two others that are essential — health and malpractice, should be provided by your employer. Remember, before purchasing any policy, talk to your colleagues; get a sense of what premiums ought to be. And always get competing bids.

Disability insurance
Your chances of becoming temporarily disabled are far greater than your chances of dying before retirement. As an employee, injuries or diseases that result from employment can be covered under workers' compensation laws. You should discuss this with your employer. Obviously not all disabilities are a result of your work, and other forms of coverage should be considered. When you are young, coverage should encompass as much of your monthly income as possible. Usually an insurance company will not cover more than 70% of your income, although some policies contain provisions for inflation. The amount of insurance necessary will also increase as your income increases and your lifestyle changes, and then it should diminish as you build your net worth and approach retirement.

It is extremely important to understand the difference in policies and not just accept one based upon the recommendations of an agent. Here are some features that you should carefully consider before selecting a policy:

(1) *Maximum benefit period*: length of time benefits will be paid in case of disability.

(2) *Perils insured against:* whether accident alone or accident and sickness.

(3) *Elimination period:* the time you must wait before disability benefits will start.

(4) *Definition of disability:* this is the most important provision. There are three common definitions: *'any occupation,' 'own occupation,'* and *'split definition.'* The 'any occupation' is the least desirable because benefits will be based upon an ability to engage in *any* fitting occupation related to education or training. Obviously then, the 'own occupation,' is the most desirable. The 'split definition' is a compromise between the other two.

Automobile insurance

In states where premiums are regulated, the only way to modify the cost is by changing the 'limits of coverage' and other types of optional coverage. In other states there can be a great difference in premiums from one company to the next. Your state insurance commissioner should be able to provide you with information on how rates are set and what options are available. For example, if you are a careful driver, raising your deductible will cut your premiums. If your car is old, you may want to drop your collision coverage. (Also, you could raise the deductible (money paid by the insured person, or out-of-pocket expense) on your medical policy if you already have health coverage). If you have had moving traffic violations, make sure that they are removed from your record after 3 years.

The one coverage that you should never cut corners on is liability. The minimal requirement in many states is not nearly enough.

If you find yourself living from paycheck to paycheck, it would be prudent to keep your old car and put off buying or leasing that fancy sports car you have been lusting after for a few more years. An expensive car will burden you with high upkeep and even higher insurance premiums.

Life insurance

This is to protect survivors against the economic risk of premature death. The proceeds paid as a result of an insured's death are exempt from income tax. The major decision here will be whether to buy *term life* insurance as opposed to one of the various forms of *whole life.*

The expression 'buy term and invest the difference' simply means that term life insurance is considerably less expensive than whole life. A disadvantage is that term gets more expensive as you get older. However, if you are successful at managing your finances, your need for life insurance should diminish with time.

Whole life insurance could be considered a hybrid because it provides not only insurance on your life, but also a method of forced savings for those who find money management difficult. Historically, these types of policies have paid very low rates of return compared to other investments, but this has improved in recent years.

As you are just starting out and you need access to your dollars, it would be inadvisable to tie up your money in a whole life policy. Annual renewable term will provide you with the least expensive, and most practical coverage.

Life insurance should not be considered a strike-it-rich lottery. Avoid purchasing more than you need. Base your decision on realistic estimates using factors such as funeral costs, the cost of raising your children (educational as well as material needs) and the needs of the surviving spouse — does he or she work? Will he or she remarry?

Homeowners insurance

There are seven basic variations of homeowners policies. It does not matter whether you own a home, a condominium, or are simply a tenant, you will need one of these policies. People who rent seem to ignore this need, with only one tenant in four having tenant's insurance, while 95% of all homeowners carry homeowner's insurance[7]. Yet their risk of loss is every bit as great.

The important provision to watch for here is *'replacement cost.'* If this provision is absent, the insurer would pay only on the basis of the value at the time of loss or *'actual cash value.'*

Again, I repeat, the cost of coverage will vary from one company to the next. *Get competitive bids.*

ESTATE, RETIREMENT AND TAX PLANNING

Volumes have been written about each of these topics. However, at this point in your career you can keep it simple, get a feel for things and then perhaps use more sophisticated strategies later on.

Estate planning

This allows for the orderly transfer of your wealth, and is important whether your estate is large or small. If your estate is modest, there are some techniques that can be used that are inexpensive and simple.

Planning adequate support for your dependents is very important, and can be accomplished with the purchase of a life insurance policy.

Holding property jointly has been referred to as the 'poor man's will.' One advantage is the avoidance in several states of the state inheritance tax. Another is the avoidance of probate court where wills and the administration of estates and related matters are dealt with. This can be time-consuming and expensive. Jointly held property is fine up to a point. However, if the decedent has any special wishes regarding the final disposition of certain property, they can be ignored by the survivor. And if children are involved, guardians must be assigned and assets managed for their benefit. This is why *every adult should have a will.*

Intestate (dying without a will) distribution is governed by the laws of each state, and can result in increased costs and delays (probate), and a court mandated distribution of an estate that was never intended by the deceased. Even a will that is poorly thought out or vague can lead to a great deal of enmity — hurt feelings, families torn apart and expensive court battles. Fashioned properly, your will is your final message on earth and leaves no questions concerning certain wishes and bequests. In it you can name an executor who has a legal duty to see to it that your final wishes are carried out, some of which might deal with items of little or no monetary value, but important to those who receive them just the same.

Certain legal requirements must be met in order to insure that your will is valid. Although generic fill-in-the-blank forms can be purchased, it is advisable to seek the counsel of an attorney. The lawyer's fee should not exceed $150–$250 for executing a pair of simple wills. He or she can also offer future advice regarding various types of trusts and how to avoid estate taxes.

Retirement planning

Although it seems a long way off, you should start considering what will be needed during retirement. This has become increasingly important because people are living longer, in many cases far beyond their age of retirement. Some of you might eventually participate in a corporate retirement program. In addition, there are other potential supplemental sources of retirement income such as Social Security retirement benefits, individual retirement account annuities, life insurance cash values and, of course, prudent investments.

Tax planning

Your objective regarding taxes is to legitimately reduce them as much as possible. Some of the taxes you have to deal with are federal and state income, sales, Social Security, local income, estate and inheritance, gift and property, just to mention a few. Tax-saving techniques that you may take advantage of in years to come are:

(1) Postponing income to another year;

(2) Shifting income to others, such as your children ; and

(3) Reducing or eliminating taxes through the use of tax deductions, exemptions and credits.

As your earnings increase, your finances will become more and more complicated, outstripping your ability to personally handle every detail. At this point you will have to give up some control and seek the services of a qualified accountant and tax attorney.

INVESTING
Paul Erdman, a famous novelist, once said, 'the entire essence of America is the hope to make money, then make money with money, then make lots of money with lots of money.'

You will benefit from that advice as long as you take your time and avoid risky get-rich-quick propositions. Remember the old adage — 'slow and steady wins the race.' Never look backward and become obsessive on all the 'if onlys' that represent missed opportunities[8].

When you have accumulated enough savings to consider avenues for your money other than a savings account or money-market fund, there are vast numbers of investments and investment strategies available, conservatively estimated at well over 100 000[9].

I could not possibly use the space in this chapter to tell you specifically where to put your money. A great many books have been written on this subject and are available in book stores and libraries. Then you must determine what suits you best. However, there is some general information and recommendations that I will share with you.

There are generally two types of investments available to the individual investor: *fixed-dollar investments* and *variable-dollar investments.* Fixed-income securities promise a predetermined amount of income in periodic installments. Some examples are corporate bonds, municipal bonds, certificates of deposit and treasury securities, etc.

The value of variable-dollar investments is affected by market pressure. Examples of these are common stocks, mutual funds and the more speculative, stock options and commodities.

Investments can be hybrids of the two and show characteristics of each, such as preferred stock. This represents equity capital, but it also pays fixed dividends.

Money market funds pool the money of numerous investors, then invest it in diversified fixed-dollar investments. Mutual funds are similar, but instead invest in diversified stocks and bonds. Mutual funds are either loaded (charge up-front commissions) or unloaded. Most money market funds are unloaded (although there are administration costs).

Whatever your investment vehicle, staying ahead of taxes and inflation is a monumental task. If, for instance, inflation averages 6% and your taxes amount to 25% of your income, then you must earn 8% on your investments just to break even. But do not feel the urgent need to take more risk than is necessary.

Every investment has some degree of risk, even those that are considered completely safe. For example, securities issued by the US Treasury are backed by the full taxing power of the federal government. There is no risk with regard to receiving your interest earnings and the return of your principal, but there is risk in the purchasing power that your interest earnings and principal will have once you actually receive them[10]. In other words, when factoring in the effects of inflation, will the purchasing power of your investment be less in the future than it is today?

In addition to interest rate risk and purchasing power risk, you must consider the market risk of stocks, real estate, and precious metals; and do not forget political risk. For instance, the latest trend in congressional tax bills is to make them retroactive, penalizing taxpayers by changing the rules in the middle of the game, making it difficult or impossible to plan ahead.

So you can see, there is a minefield out there, and the mines are planted in shifting sands, or as they say, 'things change.' But you can protect yourself by adhering to sound financial principles, and accept the fact that you will experience some setbacks, as long as they are greatly outnumbered by your successes.

CREDIT COUNSELING
If, after analyzing your finances, you discover that you need counseling, write to the National Foundation of Consumer Credit, 8701 Georgia Avenue, Silver Spring, Maryland 20910. They will send you a list of the nearest legitimate credit counselors in your area.

You can also contact the National Foundation for Consumer Credit, 1819 H Street NW, Washington DC 20006. They will refer you to their nearest Consumer Credit Counselors office (CCC), a non-profit, business-supported organization.

SUMMARY
Financial fitness can be achieved by first setting goals and objectives, and then following a predetermined plan to achieve them. This plan is initiated by recording financial information, organizing important documents and storing them in a safe place, making a balance sheet that will be the first of a series, and creating a budget to organize your household expenses.

Next, you must determine your needs in the areas of insurance, estate planning, retirement and tax planning. Finally, after you have established household spending and savings guidelines and an emergency fund of at least 6 months take-home pay, you will be ready to work out an investment strategy.

REFERENCES
1. Tucker, J. F. (1988). *Managing Your Own Money*, p. 12. (New York: Red Dembner Enterprises Corp.)
2. Lipsey, R. G., Courant, P. N., Purvis, D. D. and Steiner, P. O. (1992). *Macroeconomics*, p. 526. (New York: Harper Collins College Publishers Inc.)
3. Weinstein, G. W. (1983). *The Lifetime Book of Money Management*, p. 14. (New York: New American Library Inc.)
4. Porter, S. (1990). *Your Finances in the 1990s*, pp. v–vi. (New York: Simon and Schuster Inc.)
5. Victor, D. A. (1984). Financial planning for success. *Dent. Econ.*, **May,** 53–7
6. Weinstein, G. W. (1983). *The Lifetime Book of Money Management*, p. 29. (New York: New American Library Inc.)
7. Porter, S. (1990). *Your Finances in the 1990s*, p. 70. (New York: Simon and Schuster Inc.)
8. Vicker, R. (1987). *The Dow Jones — Irwin Guide to Retirement Planning*, p. 156. (Homewood, IL: Dow Jones–Irwin)
9. Southworth, M. M. (1986). *Money Moves: A Guide to Financial Fitness*, p. 10. (Palo Alto, CA: Turnaround Press)
10. Tucker, J. F. (1988). *Managing your Own Money*, p. 137. (New York: Red Dembner Enterprises Corp.)

15

Transition into practice

J. Escott

INTRODUCTION

The transition into practice years will be at the same time exhilarating, terrifying, frustrating and rewarding. While you will be required to apply what you learned during medical school and training, you will also be challenged on a more personal level. The work habits you develop and the ethical values you uphold in your dealings with patients, colleagues and family will determine your success as an adult and as a physician.

The structured and passive learning as a student will be replaced by the open, more independent life of a medical practitioner. The transition will challenge your integrity, reliability, inquisitiveness and personal ethics. Although many of these traits are developed in childhood, they certainly can be improved and refined in the adult years.

The transition into practice is an area about which little is known. This is an unfortunate fact because it is a situation experienced by a majority of physicians. This chapter attempts to identify the types of difficult issues you will encounter as you enter practice and offer advice on how to deal with these stresses as seen by others who have gone through this process. The last part of this chapter deals with particular areas of physician/physician and physician/patient relationships that I feel are important to the new physician.

THE TRANSITION

The stresses involved

The best summary of the stresses experienced on entering practice is in a paper by Duttera *et al.*[1] in which they surveyed 828 practicing primary care physicians who recently entered practice in Georgia. Two-thirds reported that the transition into practice was moderately or very stressful, and more than one-third noted the stress to be equal to, or greater than, that of the internship year. This is a significant conclusion because the internship is arguably one of the most stressful jobs in the American workplace.

Duttera *et al.* summarized the ten most common problems of young physicians entering practice into five broad categories. In descending order of frequency they are:

(1) Financial difficulties;

(2) Community problems;

(3) Hospital facilities;

(4) Spouse/family problems; and

(5) Geography.

Knowing these potentially stressful areas may help direct the new practitioner into developing appropriate coping strategies. For example, one-half of the respondents in this study cited a practicing physician as their principal source of coping strategies. Training programs appeared to be less useful as only 11% of respondents reported that they were a major method of help. A disappointing 18% felt there was no source of help at all with this transition. Some groups have reported that while alarming symptoms of stress appear during this transition, there are also effective coping strategies[2]. The two most effective adaptation mechanisms included establishing good support systems with loved ones and with professional colleagues.

Personality and type of practice

Given that the level of stress is so high during the transition to practice, is there a way to know if we are entering the right type of practice? Several studies have looked at factors on career choice and do shed some light on this issue.

Weil and Schleiter[3], in their 1981 study, looked at interest in primary care vs. subspecialty medicine and predicting interest in academic medicine or clinical practice. They showed that personal variables like religion, personality and control over working conditions had greater predictive power than environmental variables (e.g. residency or the medical school attended) when choosing primary care vs. subspecialty practice and clinical practice vs. academic medicine. The major personal variable for the type of practice selected was control over working conditions (i.e. autonomy). The next most important variable was the type of medical school attended (i.e. a school that preferred students interested in primary care rather than one that preferred students oriented to research and teaching).

Duttera's five broad categories of problem areas in the transition to private practice bear out the findings of Weil and Schleiter in that four of the five categories (financial, community, family and geography) represent control over working conditions.

Practice selection was also determined very much by personality variables, as shown in a study of residents at the University of California at Los Angeles[4]. This study looked at 'patient-oriented residents' vs. 'disease-oriented residents' and found that the former evaluate their work and social environments differently from those residents that are less patient oriented. The study suggests two orientations toward medical work and careers. The patient-oriented residents are physicians who feel a great deal of pressure from the volume of knowledge they must master. They experience more physical, psychological and social distress, and are less confident. They have benevolent interpersonal needs which do not seem to be met through work. They experience lower job satisfaction and look forward to a practice interaction where they can develop long-term relationships with their patients. These physicians are more likely to enter private practice than subspecialty or academic medicine.

The disease-oriented residents are physicians who experience less pressure from the volume of knowledge to be learned, are more confident and experience less distress. They are less likely to value getting to know their patients and prefer dealing with disease. Generally, they plan to pursue subspecialty training and do not plan to enter private practice.

A patient-oriented resident may benefit from the findings in study of psychiatrists which showed that building self-confidence and relieving stress can be accomplished by forming interpersonal relationships and support systems with loved one or colleagues[2].

Practice and choices

Barbakow and Weinberger studied *Factors in Practice Location* for graduates of Alabama's primary care residents in 1980[5]. They found four factors as the most important variables in practice location. They were: acceptability of location to the spouse; availability of adequate hospital facilities; quality of the educational system; and lifestyle.

Another study compared practice patterns and stresses of male and female Harvard graduates from 1967 to 1977[6]. They made several observations:

(1) Over one-half of both men and women changed their plans regarding both field of practice and style of practice during their training. Marriage and family responsibilities were cited as reasons for the change by one-third of women.

(2) Female physicians most often reported having full-time housekeepers, while male physicians reported that their spouse took care of the children alone, or in combination with the husband or baby-sitter, 88% of the time.

(3) Female physicians were more likely than male physicians (58% vs. 38%) to report conflicts relating to marriage and family responsibilities. The most frequent conflict reported by women was that related to dual career issues. Women reported continuing in challenging and complex careers, even when they had to juggle child care.

(4) Geographic mobility was most often determined by the husband's career.

(5) Both men and women chose to keep family size small.

(6) Nearly one-half of the men and one-third of the women found resources present to help integrate career and family.

This section has attempted to give an overview of some of the issues surrounding the initial entrance to practice. While there are few scientific papers written about the transition to practice, there are a number of useful monographs on the subject. One directed to entry to private practice is particularly useful[7]. The following sections deal with some specific problem areas for new physicians.

DEALING WITH COLLEAGUES

Interpersonal relationships

This becomes increasingly important as you enter your practice years. As house officers, you will see the total range of physician interactions. Some of these will be very cordial and mutually supportive, while others hostile and destructive. For example, inappropriate comments about your colleagues may lead to a malpractice suit. Consider physicians that make statements to other doctors or lay persons about their colleagues such as: 'It's malpractice to...' or 'Why didn't he do...' Instead of making provocative and negative comments when you disagree with a particular treatment regimen, use positive statements like, 'Another way to approach this problem is...' or 'there are good and bad points to this approach...' The key is to be non-judgmental in statements made to patients and their families about other physicians. A non-critical approach to other doctors' practice also makes medical sense. For the most part, doctors make reasonable decisions based on the facts and standard of practice available to them at the time. As you were not there at the time of medical decision-making, it is very difficult to find fault (unless, of course, you are a subspecialist in the area and an expert witness). My advice is to know as much about current medical practice as you can and take care of your patients as if they were family members. This is a big enough job without being critical of others.

Consultations

Another difficult area of physician interaction is over consultations. This can be a particular problem for physicians first entering practice. Consider, for example, the curbside consultation. Remember how as house officers/ students you appreciated the consultant who would give you the pearls of diagnosis and treatment in the elevator or cafeteria, saving you effort but costing the consultant their time? Now that you are the consultant you may be tempted to say 'write me a consultation' because of financial considerations. This behavior can be perceived as arrogant and may cut you out of future referrals. The consultant who gives generously of his expertise in the cafeteria is likely to get the greatest share of referrals on the hospital wards because he/she was available and has engendered good relationships with the other staff.

Not consulting enough is the opposite problem. You have just spent 3–5 years in postgraduate residency training. You are board certified or board eligible and know how to treat 'X' disease. You get a patient with 'X' disease and, as usually happens, he is not following the classic course of the disease. Instead of asking for help, you want to prove that you can care for the patient yourself without outside help. This type of behavior is not only a potential medicolegal problem but it also cheats the patient. The smart practitioner will ask for a consultation. Two things can happen — both good. First, the consultant will likely say you are doing everything that should be done and it makes you look good. Second, the consultant offers a piece of advice that you may have overlooked. The patient is pleased that you got the appropriate help and you learned something for the next case. Seeking consultation neither makes you look bad nor does it suggest that you cannot handle a problem. Appropriate consultation demonstrates that the physican is secure and confident enough in his or her patient management to ask for a second opinion. Health care is a team effort that you want to control rather than have it control you. Sophisticated patients are very much aware of these issues and may even initiate an effort for a second opinion.

ASSUMING ADULT RESPONSIBILITY

Now that you have finished your postgraduate training program, you have to throw away the resident-student/learner approach that you have used for the last two decades for the teacher/attending/specialist approach to learning and practicing. This transition carries both desirable and undesirable points.

Autonomy and responsibility

You have the privilege of setting your own schedule and greater freedom for deciding diagnostic and therapeutic options, but you also have the obligation of doing what is right for the patient. Students/learners tend to want to use all the new procedures, tests and medications they read about. Teachers/attending physicians must take a more critical approach and weigh the benefits and risks much more closely. Many of the options you might have tried as a resident on an empirical basis may need to be discarded as you assume total responsibility for patient care and outcomes. As the attending physician, you may have to face the family when a patient needs a chest tube because an aggressive resident has caused a pneumothorax during a thoracentesis. A consistently known outcome is better than initiating procedures and treatments based on possible benefits but with a higher risk of complication.

Limitations

You need to know your limitations as a practitioner. As a responsible adult medical practitioner you must be honest with yourself and critically evaluate what you can and cannot do. A procedure performed only twice a year may be better and more safely carried out by a consultant, with or without your help. A disease you rarely see may be better treated by a consultant, again with or without your help. Ironically, once you are in a private practice, you are the best judge of your limitations. You must be prepared to practice according to those limitations and do what is best for your patients.

BUILDING A PRACTICE

It is well known that there are several As to success in practice. These recommendations apply to any person in a small business that must deal with sophisticated consumers. They are, in order of importance: availability, affability, ability and, in recent years, affordability.

Availability

It is a simple fact that the more available you are, the busier you will be. A former partner of mine once said, 'Your first year in practice, you answer your phone each time it rings.' You also must call patients back promptly. Sick patients deserve your expertise in a timely manner.

Be available to the emergency department. Emergency rooms are looking for doctors to accept patients who have no personal physician of their own. If they cannot get hold of you, you will not get the patient — and if this happens often, they will no longer bother to call you again. Many physicians who take Wednesday afternoon off to play golf lose patients to physicians who are in the office at that time. In addition, with both spouses working, many families need physicians with evening and/or Saturday hours. While no one can be available all the time, it is up to you to determine what level of availability you are willing to provide. The more time you are available for patient care, the more patients and doctors will consult with you.

Affability

This applies to dealing with patients and colleagues alike. The physician who is always courteous and friendly will get more referrals, consults and patients than one who is irritable and hostile when called. Patients and doctors like to consult with approachable, friendly, non-critical colleagues.

Included under being affable is being appropriately dressed. Years of discussions with residents concerning dress code has taught me that people will dress as they see fit. Some dress opposite the dress code in order to demonstrate their individuality. Now that you are on your own, take a closer look at your dress. Part of being affable is to be appealing to your patients and colleagues. John T. Molloy, the dress for success expert, recommends that doctors wear sport coats rather than classic cut suits as they make us look approachable and less threatening to patients[8]. Although wearing a tie is a sign of authority in our society, you do not have to look like a banker. If you want to increase your credibility and enhance your mature image, wear clean, well fitted and conservative clothes. Patients are in need of your brain, not the clothes on your back.

Ability

Your skill as a physician is of great importance. All of the above traits are worthless if you are a poor physician. Use self-directed study (see Chapter 11) and continuing medical education (CME) to keep yourself current. Your medical knowledge is at its peak when you leave your training program. Now you are on your own, read and talk to your colleagues about new treatments and procedures. Attend CME courses and workshops to help you acquire new skills. Reviewing the literature and being critical of what you read are skills you learned as residents and will use as a primary learning tool after you leave training. One good way to keep abreast of new developments in your field is to choose one journal in that area which is comprehensive, well written, current and critical. Try to read that one journal thoroughly every month. Then pick up other articles of interest as they surface. A planned approach like this will help keep you current in your field. One look at someone's stack of unread journals shows you the fallacy of trying to read too much or not having a selective, organized approach. The ability to critically and efficiently review current literature is a skill of most successful practitioners. Listening to cassette tapes in your car is also very efficient and productive (see Chapter 11).

Affordability

A major issue in the 1990s is the cost of medical care. You have seen the rise of managed care and efforts are under way to get some type of health insurance for everyone. Physician fees are being monitored and regulated as never before. Being affordable means not only a fee structure in line with other physicians, but also choosing the right managed care plans for your practice. Although a thorough discussion of fees is beyond the scope of this book it is well to remember sound economic principles. In a free market a better product or service commands a higher fee. In a controlled market such as a health maintenance organization, outstanding service will eventually result in a higher salary.

SUMMARY
The transition to practice requires a complex combination of knowledge and workplace skills. Knowledge, hard work and honesty form the framework for success in medicine or any other profession.

REFERENCES
1. Duttera, M. J., Hummel, G. R., Brown, E. E. and Miller, H. M. (1983). Entry into practice: problems in making the transition. *J. Fam. Pract.,* **17,** 529–31
2. Looney, J. G., Harding, R. K., Blotcky, M. J. and Barnhart, F. D. (1980). Psychiatrist's transition from training to career: stress and mastery. *Am. J. Psychiatry,* **137,** 32–6
3. Weil, P. A. and Schleitel, M. K. (1981). National study of internal medicine manpower: VI. Factors predicting preferences of residents for careers in primary care or subspeciality care and clinical practice or academic medicine. *Ann. Intern. Med.,* **94,** 691–703
4. Linn, L. S. (1981). Career orientations and the quality of working life among medical interns and residents. *Soc. Sci. Med.,* **15A,** 259–63
5. Barbakow, P. and Weinberger, D. (1981). Factors in practice location. *J. Med. Assoc. State of Alabama,* **51,** 48–54
6. Nedelson, C. C., Notman, M. T. and Lowenstein, P. (1979). The practice pattern, life styles, and stresses of women and men entering medicine: a follow-up study of Harvard Medical School graduates from 1967 to 1977. *J. Am. Med. Assoc.,* **34,** 400–6
7. McCue, J. D. and Ficalora, R. D. (1991). *Private Practice: A Guide to Getting Started.* (Boston: Little, Brown and Co.)
8. Molloy, J. T. (1988). *New Dress for Success.* (New York: Warner Books)

Index